Fascial Manipulation®
– Stecco® method
The practitioner's perspective

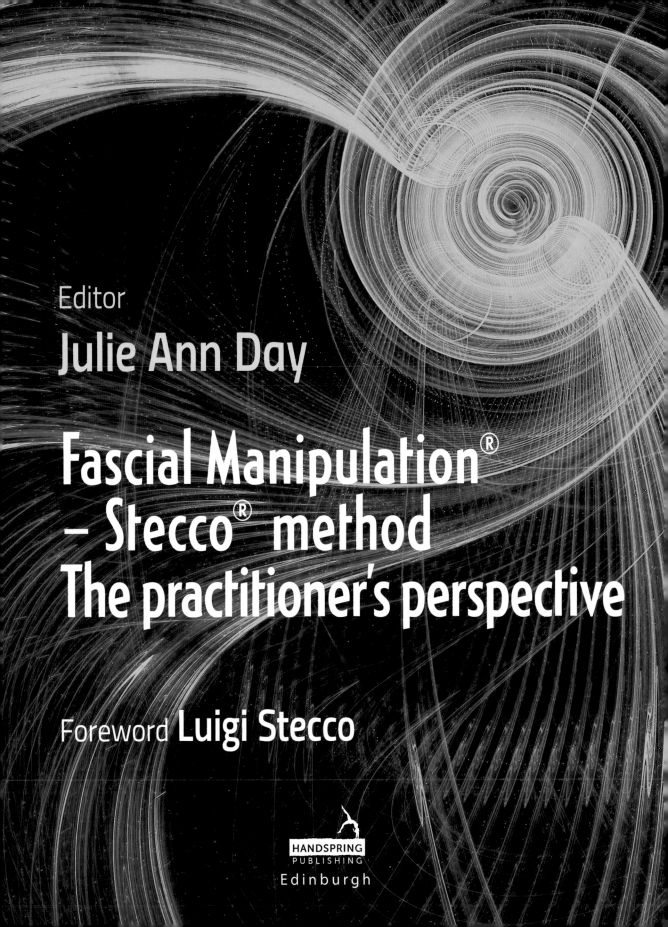

Editor

Julie Ann Day

Fascial Manipulation®
– Stecco® method
The practitioner's perspective

Foreword **Luigi Stecco**

HANDSPRING
PUBLISHING
Edinburgh

HANDSPRING PUBLISHING LIMITED
The Old Manse, Fountainhall,
Pencaitland, East Lothian
EH34 5EY, Scotland
Tel: +44 1875 341 859
Website: www.handspringpublishing.com

First published 2018 in the United Kingdom by Handspring Publishing

ISBN 978-1-912085-01-9

British Library Cataloguing in Publication Data
A catalogue record for this book is available from the British Library

Library of Congress Cataloguing in Publication Data
A catalog record for this book is available from the Library of Congress

Notice
Neither the Publisher nor the Author assumes any responsibility for any loss or injury and/or damage to persons or property arising out of or relating to any use of the material contained in this book. It is the responsibility of the treating practitioner, relying on independent expertise and knowledge of the patient, to determine the best treatment and method of application for the patient.

Commissioning Editor Mary Law
Developmental Editor Andrew Stevenson
Project Manager Barbara McAviney
Copy-editor Stephanie Pickering
Designer Bruce Hogarth
Indexer Aptara corp, India
Typesetter DiTech, India
Printer Melita, Malta

The
Publisher's
policy is to use
paper manufactured
from sustainable forests

CONTENTS

ACKNOWLEDGMENTS

I would like to thank all of the contributors to this book for sharing their invaluable know-how and experience.

Special thanks to Mary Law from Handspring Publishing, for encouraging me to undertake this journey and supporting me step-by-step along the way, and to the rest of the fantastic Handspring team for their generous ongoing guidance.

I particularly wish to thank Luigi Stecco, both for sharing some of his private letters and, above all, for his inspiring passion, the driving force behind all my fascial adventures.

I am also infinitely grateful to my partner, Sergio, who has kept me nourished with his delicious Italian cooking and his wise words of encouragement throughout the whole editing process.

Julie Day

Copyright notice – illustrations

CONTRIBUTORS

Marco Branchini PT, MS, Bologna, Italy
Faculty member and Didactic Coordinator of
Physiotherapy degree course, University of Bologna.
Senior Fascial Manipulation® teacher. Founding member
of Fascial Manipulation Association.

Natalie Brettler BPT, Tel Aviv, Israel
Private practitioner. Team physiotherapist for Israel's
national team of rhythmic gymnastics. Fascial
Manipulation® teacher.

Jaroslaw Ciechomski PT, PhD, DO, Poznan, Poland
Private practitioner and director of Aktiv Osteopathy
and Rehabilitation clinic, Poznan, Poland. Senior Fascial
Manipulation® teacher. Editor-in-chief of 'Practical
Physiotherapy and Rehabilitation' journal.

Lorenzo Copetti PT, Tolmezzo, Italy
Private practitioner, Senior Fascial Manipulation®
teacher. Founding member of Fascial Manipulation
Association. Former University of Udine faculty member.

Julie Ann Day PT, Padova, Italy
Azienda ULSS 6 Euganea, Padova. Senior Fascial
Manipulation® teacher. Founding member of Fascial
Manipulation Association.

Lorenzo Freschi PT Cesena, Italy
Private practitioner. Former team physiotherapist for
Cesena male basketball team. Fascial Manipulation for
Internal Dysfunctions (FMID) teacher.

Warren I. Hammer DC, MS, DABCO, Norwalk (CT), USA
Postgraduate Faculty of New York Chiropractic College.
Author of 'Functional Soft-Tissue Examination and
Treatment by Manual Methods' (3rd edn, 2007), Fascial
Manipulation® teacher.

Tiina Lahtinen-Suopanki Senior PT, OMT, Helsinki,
Finland
Private practitioner at Rehabilitation Center Orton,
Helsinki. Lecturer for Finnish Association of Orthopedic
Manual Therapy and Finnish Physiotherapy Association.
Fascial Manipulation® teacher.

Angela Mackenzie RMT, Chilliwack, BC, Canada
Member of College of Massage Therapists of British
Columbia and Massage Therapists' Association of BC,

Canada. Owner of Rebound to Health clinic, Chilliwack,
BC, Canada.

Eran Mangel BPT, Tel Aviv, Israel
Co-founder, owner and Head of Physiotherapy
Department at Medix, Tel Aviv. Former team
physiotherapist for Israel's national handball and women
and men's basketball teams.

Cheryl Megalos BScPT, CGIMS, Vancouver, Canada
Private practitioner, Westside Physiotherapy and Hand
clinic, Vancouver, BC. Fascial Manipulation® teacher.
Member of the Canadian Physiotherapy Association and
the Fascial Manipulation Association.

Stephen F. Oswald DO, New York, USA
Private practitioner. Fascial Manipulation® teacher.
Member of the Fascial Manipulation Association.
Member of the Fascial Research Society.

Andrea Pasini PT, Cesena, Italy
Private practitioner. Fascial Manipulation for Internal
Dysfunctions (FMID) teacher. Member of the Fascial
Manipulation Association.

Larry Steinbeck PT, MSc Phys Ed, CMTPT, Atlanta, USA
Manager of Physical Therapy at Atlanta Falcons Physical
Therapy Center/Jasper Physical Therapy, GA, USA.
Fascial Manipulation® teacher. Faculty member for
Myopain Seminars®, Bethesda, MD.

Hitoshi Takei PT, PhD, OMPT, FMT, GPTH.O.I, Tokyo,
Japan
Faculty of Health Sciences Division of Physical Therapy,
Tokyo Metropolitan University. Member of International
Federation of Orthopedic Manual Physical Therapists
Association (IFOMPT). Fascial Manipulation® teacher.

Nita Tolvanen BPT, Helsinki, Finland
Advanced Specialist in Pediatric Physiotherapy (Neuro-
Developmental-Treatment/Bobath approach) at
Terapiakeskus Terapeija center, Vantaa, Finland.

Colleen Whiteford PT, DPT, OCS, CMTPT, New Market,
Virginia, USA
Private practitioner, Co-owner of Appalachian Physical
Therapy, Inc. Faculty member for Myopain Seminars®,
Bethesda, MD.

FOREWORD

In the foreword to this new book, proposed and edited by Julie Ann Day, I would like to talk about my experiences at the beginning of my career as a physiotherapist because they may well be similar to those described by the various authors who have contributed to this text.

In Italy, in the 1970s, rehabilitation consisted mostly of active or passive exercises and electrotherapy. Whenever I was treating a patient I felt like I was merely performing pre-determined protocols and did not feel that I was particularly contributing to their recovery. Results with regards to the patients' dysfunctions were disappointing and my satisfaction was minimal. The working hours just never seemed to pass.

Nevertheless, I aspired to be the protagonist of my work and I wanted to use my hands to reduce the suffering of others. To achieve this goal, I studied the various manual therapy methods that were available at that time, extrapolating ideas from each one to develop the indications that have culminated in the Fascial Manipulation® (FM) method. Working with this method fueled my own enthusiasm and the days were suddenly too short to be able to treat all of the patients that were seeking care. At the end of each day, I often thought about the cases I had treated. While I was pleased with those that had been resolved, I interrogated myself about why I had not been able to resolve others.

The desire to provide explanations for both the successes and the failures in my work impelled me to seek out all the information I could find in anatomical texts regarding the fascia and its connections. As my studies advanced, the marvelous architecture of the fascia began to take shape for me. I realized that it was not just a tissue that was merely filling spaces but it was the actual heart and soul of movement, coordinating it and collaborating with the central and autonomic nervous systems.

With FM some musculoskeletal dysfunctions that had previously required up to 10 physiotherapy treatments improved significantly in a single session. In 1986, these results encouraged me to write down my experiences in my very first booklet. I was motivated by the idea of sharing the potential of this new manual therapy with my colleagues. I feel certain that this is the same type of motivation that has inspired Julie to gather together these testimonials from colleagues who have been practicing this method for a number of years. Therefore, I am extremely grateful to all of these colleagues for their contribution to spreading the knowledge of a method that is decisive for resolving many musculoskeletal and internal dysfunctions.

Luigi Stecco PT
Creator of Fascial Manipulation®–Stecco® method
Private practitioner, Arzignano (VI), Italy
Co-founder of the Fascial Manipulation
Institute, Padova, Italy
2018

PREFACE

When I first met Luigi Stecco, in Milan in 1991, we were both attending a weekend course called 'Fascia, blood and pulsology', based on the Danis Bois method. Stecco had brought with him a suitcase full of copies of his second self-published book and was earnestly seeking out interested colleagues with whom he could discuss his ideas about fascia. Over pizza that evening he explained the basics of his concepts. As an Australian trained physiotherapist I was fascinated by Stecco's ability to expand on the anatomy of fascia and its relationship to acupuncture, neurology, and motor control. However, I came away from that encounter having understood perhaps only 15 per cent of what he was talking about! At the same time I was convinced that he was onto something quite special. We kept in touch over the following years and from time to time I translated some short letters for him. These letters that were mostly addressed to pain and soft-tissue experts in different countries. However, it was not until 1998 that I had my first opportunity to attend a course held by Luigi Stecco. Since then I have become progressively involved in the organizational, translational, and didactical aspects related to this method.

A teacher of Fascial Manipulation®–Stecco® method (Level I and II) since 2003, I have translated four of Stecco's texts from Italian to English, two of which have recently gone to second editions. Developing new, method-specific terms in English presented a significant challenge but it also forced me to analyze Stecco's words with great attention. Not an easy author to translate, Stecco assumes that his reader has a vast knowledge of comparative anatomy and fascia and, rather than suggesting hypotheses, he has the tendency to make outright statements. This presented a further challenge in staying true to his word without sounding too presumptuous. However, since that first encounter in 1991, my understanding of the human fascial system has continued to be nurtured and this knowledge is now an integral part of my ongoing clinical work as a physiotherapist.

Through my teaching work I have had the pleasure of meeting and studying with an international group of practitioners, all of whom were already well-established in their own fields when they first encountered Stecco's model and method. This diverse group (physiotherapists, chiropractors, osteopaths, medical doctors, and massage therapists) had successful practices, and some also had reputable teaching and research careers, both locally and internationally.

The intention of this book is to give a voice to some of these professionals who, without any particular need to adopt a completely new paradigm, approached this new model from an analytical position. While different studies have now examined the efficacy of this method (Picelli et al. 2011; Branchini et al. 2016; Busato et al. 2016), a substantial body of published clinical research was lacking in the initial stages. Nevertheless, the clinical results they witnessed by applying this model convinced them to explore this method further, integrating it into their clinical work. The contributors to this book are representative of many others who have adopted this new paradigm for musculoskeletal and visceral dysfunctions. Collectively, their feedback and enthusiasm have encouraged me to continue delving into the Stecco® method, up to the present day and into the future.

I hope that, by presenting case examples contributed from such a wide range of experienced professionals, this book will encourage others to consider incorporating Fascial Manipulation®–Stecco® method into their everyday clinical practice.

Julie Ann Day, Physiotherapist,
Azienda ULSS 6 Euganea,
Padova, Italy
Senior Fascial Manipulation® teacher
Founding member of Fascial Manipulation
Association and ex-member of the Executive Council
January 2018

PREFACE *continued*

References

Branchini M, Lopopolo F, Andreoli E, Loreti I, Marchand AM and Stecco A (2016) Fascial Manipulation® for chronic aspecific low back pain: A single blinded randomized controlled trial. F1000 Research 4: 1208.

Busato M, Quagliati C, Magri L, Filippi A, Sanna A, Branchini M, Marchand AM and Stecco A (2016) Fascial manipulation associated with standard care compared to only standard postsurgical care for total hip arthroplasty: A randomized controlled trial. PM & R 8(12): 1142–50.

Picelli A, Ledro G, Turrina A, Stecco C, Santilli V and Smania N (2011) Effects of myofascial technique in patients with subacute whiplash associated disorders: A pilot study. European Journal of Physical and Rehabilitation Medicine 47(4): 561–8.

GLOSSARY

Terminology for musculoskeletal model

Center of coordination CC Stretch generated from contraction of the intrafusal fibers of muscle spindles causes the activation of motor units that are involved in a specific direction of movement. The subsequent vectors produced converge in the CC, which is a specific point of the epimysial fascia within each myofascial unit.

Center of fusion CF Small areas of fascia located over retinacula and around joints that monitor movements in intermediate directions between two planes, and movements of adjacent segments in different directions. CFs are linked either by longitudinal collagen fibers to form myofascial diagonals or via obliquely orientated collagen fibers to form myofascial spirals.

Center of perception CP An area around the joint of the myofascial unit where tension exerted on the insertional tendon by the extrafusal fibers of the myofascial unit converges.

Directions of movement Stecco uses new terminology to describe movement in terms of directions on the three spatial planes. All forward movements on a sagittal plane are called *antemotion* and all backward movements *retromotion*. Adduction and abduction are substituted by *lateromotion* (from the center to the periphery) and *mediomotion* (from the periphery to the center), and *intrarotation* and *extrarotation* are used when movement occurs on the horizontal plane. Thus, the mf (myofascial) units of antemotion and retromotion govern movements on the sagittal plane, the mf units of lateromotion and mediomotion govern movements on the frontal (coronal) plane and the mf units of intrarotation and extrarotation govern movements on the horizontal plane.

Densification The aponeurotic fascia is formed by layers of dense connective tissue interposed by loose connective tissue, which allows for gliding. Densification involves an increase in viscosity of the hyaluronan component within the extracellular matrix of this loose connective tissue and it has the potential to alter the physiology of the fasciae.

Myofascial sequences, mf sequence Longitudinal collagen fibers connect unidirectional mf (myofascial) units together to form myofascial sequences (mf sequence). A single mf sequence synchronizes the movement of body segments in one direction on one plane. There are six mf sequences: antemotion and retromotion (sagittal plane); lateromotion and mediomotion (frontal plane); intrarotation and extrarotation (horizontal plane).

Myofascial unit, mf unit Each mf unit consists of motor units involved in carrying out movement in a single direction, tendons that transmit the forces of these motor units, the joint that is moved and the fascia that surrounds all of the above structures. The name of each mf unit is formed by the direction of movement plus the segment that is moved, e.g., retromotion lumbi (re-lu), backward movement of the lumbar segment on the sagittal plane.

Myofascial spiral, mf spiral Centers of fusion connected by spiral form collagen fibers that follow an anatomically traceable spiral pathway along limbs and either across or around the trunk.

Terminology for internal dysfunctions model

Apparatus Internal apparatus is distributed throughout the trunk and connected via apparatus–fascial sequences extending along the anterior and posterior trunk walls. Tensional compensations originating from the fasciae of the trunk and the internal fasciae can spread to the limbs and the head, and tension originating from the limbs and the head can interfere with the peristalsis of the internal apparatus.

Apparatus–fascial sequences, a-f sequences There are three apparatus-fascial sequences in the trunk: (1) visceral sequence, formed by the pleura and peritoneum (respiratory and digestive apparatus); (2) vascular sequence, located in the retroperitoneal region (circulatory and urinary apparatus); (3) glandular sequence, which includes the endocrine and hematopoietic apparatus. If fascial densification extends to include a number of trunk segments (i.e., along a catenary), it affects a chain of extramural ganglia and dysfunction can involve one or more apparatus.

Catenary The union of the three tensile structures of the trunk (TH, LU, and PV) into a single, longitudinal tensile structure aligns each tensor along the line of greatest tension or catenary. Catenaries can be categorized as anteroposterior, latero-lateral, and oblique and each catenary is related to a chain of extramural ganglia. Each single catenary is sustained distally by tensors located in the limbs (see Distal tensors).

Distal tensors Centers of fusion in the extremities: ankle, foot, wrist, and hands, that represent the distal parts of the catenaries.

Fascial Manipulation for Internal Dysfunctions
FMID Based on a specific model for internal fasciae, this approach acts on the fasciae of the trunk wall and its tensors in order to eliminate any interference between the abdominal canister and the peristalsis of its contents that may be causing visceral dysfunctions.

Investing fasciae The thin, elastic, and very well innervated visceral fasciae that are closely related to the individual organ, giving shape to it and supporting the parenchyma.

Insertional fasciae The thick fibrous sheets – less elastic, less innervated, but containing larger and myelinated nerves – that form compartments for the organs and also connect the internal organs to the musculoskeletal system.

Organ–fascial units, o-f units Each o-f unit consists of organs involved in the same function and located within the same body cavity, the internal fascia that connects these synergic organs together, and the intramural neuronal network and the intramural autonomic ganglia that synchronize these organs. According to their function, they can be divided into visceral, vascular, or glandular o-f units.

Pivot points Fixed anchorage points, formed bones and joints around shoulder and pelvic girdles located along catenaries; called pivot points because they allow the body to continuously readjust its tensional alignment.

Superficial fascia quadrants When the superficial fascia is analyzed in transversal and longitudinal directions, it can be divided into quadrants. Each quadrant is innervated by a specific cutaneous nerve. The letter 'q' placed before the area of the quadrant distinguishes it from a diagonal.

Systems The role of the systems is to maintain homeostasis and they are connected with the hypodermis, which includes the superficial fascia. They involve three systems connected with the external environment (cutaneous, adipose, and lymphatic) and three internal systems (thermoregulatory, metabolic, and immune), which are all disseminated throughout the body in a uniform manner and are related to macroscopic paravertebral and prevertebral ganglia.

Tensile structures In FMID, each segment of the trunk is considered as a cylinder in which the elastic anterior trunk wall, together with the more rigid posterior wall, form a tensile structure. If fascial densification involves a trunk wall tensor of a single tensile structure, then activity of the intramural ganglia can be affected and peristalsis of an o-f unit within that tensile structure can become dysfunctional.

INTRODUCTION
Julie Ann Day

The Fascial Manipulation®–Stecco® (FM) method is a manual method for the treatment of fascial dysfunction and myofascial pain. Developed by Italian physiotherapist Luigi Stecco, it is based on a new interpretation of the musculo-skeletal and internal fasciae systems that places fasciae in a proactive role. This new model has been adopted by a growing number of professionals from different fields of manual therapy, such as physiotherapy, chiropractic, medicine, osteopathy, and massage therapy. This book reports the experiences of some of these professionals, all of whom were well established in their own fields when they first encountered this method. The case reports, opinions, and clinical reasoning presented by them will be valuable for colleagues who are beginning to use this method as well as for other professionals who are curious about its application.

How did the Fascial Manipulation®–Stecco® method begin?

The development of FM dates back to the early 1970s, when Luigi Stecco first became fascinated by the popularity of local 'bonesetters' in the rural area of northern Italy where he grew up. As a student of physiotherapy, Stecco was frustrated because these 'bonesetters,' who had had no formal training, were unable to explain their clinical results in anatomical and physiological terms.

As a physiotherapist (since 1973), Stecco began wide-ranging investigations in an effort to explain the effectiveness of these vigorous soft tissue treatments. He delved into aspects of osteopathy, relaxation techniques, postural exercises, connective tissue massage by Elizabeth Dicke, the approach of Dr James Cyriax, acupuncture, and Janet Travell's trigger points. The clinical results he obtained by applying these methods were promising. However, it was not until he was introduced to Ida Rolf's work (through Italian translations of Leon Chaitow's publications) that he realized that joints can be made to work better by modifying the connective tissue surrounding the muscles known as fascia. Thus, he began to study everything he could find that addressed this tissue, gleaning information about fascial connections from sources including anatomy and comparative anatomy texts, as well as the works of Marcel Bienfait and the kinetic chains described by Françoise Mézières, until he was able to trace a relationship between acupuncture meridians and these kinetic chains.

After more than 10 years of individual study and clinical work, Stecco first published his proposals concerning the human fascial system in 1987 (Figure I.1).

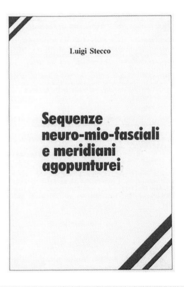

Figure I.1
Cover of the first Italian-language book concerning the human fascial system published by Luigi Stecco in 1987. Courtesy of Luigi Stecco

In this self-funded booklet, entitled 'Sequenze neuro-mio-fasciali e meridiani agopunturei' (in English: 'Myofascial sequences and acupuncture meridians'), Stecco proposed that deep friction over specific points on muscle bellies could loosen muscular fascia, thereby freeing embedded nerve endings, and that traceable myofascial sequences had numerous correlations to acupuncture meridians. At first, this publication did not receive much attention from his Italian peers. Unperturbed, Stecco sought out confirmation from further afield. As mentioned in the editor's Preface, he was corresponding with other experts, including the likes of David G. Simons, Professor H. Heine from Witten/Herdecke University (Figure I.2) and also Dr Karl Lewitt from Prague.

DAVID G. SIMONS, M.D.
324 12th Street
Huntington Beach, CA 92648-4519
United States of America
Telephone: (714) 969-1235

7 April 1987

Luigi Stecco
Via Piacenza, 3
Arzignano, 36-71
(Vicenza) Italy

Dear Mr. Stecco:

My apologies for this delayed response to your letters of 11 January and 14 February 1987. I do not speak and I do not read Italian. My first attempt to find someone to translate your letters came to nothing.

From your letters and the illustrations in the manuscript, I have the impression that you are relating myofascial trigger points in some way to acupuncture (acupressure) points. You also make the statement that research and documentation are scanty. The last is, fortunately, not the case.

I think of myofascial trigger points as being something quite different from, and basically totally independent of, acupuncture points. It is not surprising that some acupuncture points may coincide with trigger points considering how acupuncture (acupressure) points are sometimes located by finding areas of tenderness.

Meanwhile, I will ask the person who translated your letters to try to find exactly what your hypotheses is from your manuscript.

For your information, I am enclosing a list of current research relating to myofascial trigger points that may be of help to you. I am also enclosing a reprint of a Letter to the Editor of PAIN describing the cause of myofascial trigger points that is now being proven correct by research.

The basic document describing trigger points is, of course, THE TRIGGER POINT MANUAL (brochure enclosed). I understand it is being translated into Italian and should be available in Italy before too much longer. It was due to be published by Giorgio Ghendini in the first quarter of 1987 based on information from one year ago.

Very sincerely yours,

David G. Simons, M.D.

DGS/bz
Enc.

UNIVERSITÄT WITTEN/HERDECKE
MEDIZINISCHE FAKULTÄT

Via Oberdan 81
91025 Marsala (TP)

Medizinische Fakultät · Alfred-Herrhausen-Str. 50 · 58448 Witten

Dr. Luigi Stecco
Via Piacenza 3, Arzignano

I - 36071 Vicenza

Anatomisches und Klinisch-Morphologisches Institut
Institutsleiter
Prof.Dr.rer.nat.med.habil. Hartmut Heine
Tel. 0 23 02 / 926-0
Tel. 0 23 02 / 926-724
Fax 0 23 02 / 926-407

Witten, 14.5.96
Hei/He

Dear Colleague,

many thanks for your highly scientific and interesting book „La manipolazione neuroconnectivale".

You have done an analytical masterwork. The functional myo-fascial interactions corresponding to myo-tendinous kinetic chains indeed have the same direction as acupuncture meridians. The acupuncture points as fascia perforating nerve-vessel bundles wrapped in loose connective tissue must be irritated by each myo-fascial motion. I think one of the most important reactions within an acupuncture point are axon-reflexes which can continue along the myofascial chains from point to point as you have described it (compare *Zhang* 1996). In this respect your findings on coordination centres will be of strong interest.

In Vienna Dozent Dr. med. Otto *Bergsmann* has described meridians as musculo-tendinous chains but has not looked to the fascia (*Bergsmann*, O. und R. *Bergsmann*: Projektionssymptome. Facultas Verlag, Wien 1988, ISBN Nr. 3-85076-238-6).

Your work will be a great stimulus for investigations in all kind of rheumatical diseases.

I congratulate you to this work and remain

Sincerely yours

(Prof. Dr. H. Heine)

Private Universität Witten/Herdecke GmbH
Geschäftsführer: Dr. Konrad Schily (Präsident), Dr. Bernd Kümmel (Vizepräsident), Dipl.-Kfm. Bernhard Stöhr (kaufm.)
Sitz der Gesellschaft: Witten · Amtsgericht Witten HRB 703
Bankkonten: Deutsche Bank AG Witten (BLZ 430 700 61) Kto.-Nr. 8 327 777 · Stadtsparkasse Witten (BLZ 452 500 35) Kto.-Nr. 10 900

Figure I.2
Examples of letters to Luigi Stecco from David Simons and Professor H. Heine. Private letters, courtesy of Luigi Stecco

David G. Simons then invited him to present a poster at the First International Symposium on Myofascial Pain and Fibromyalgia that was held in Minneapolis (USA) in 1989 (Figure I.3).

In this poster, Stecco argued that these key fascial points, which he called *centers of coordination*, represented the convergence point of the vectors formed by various muscular forces operating on a segment of fascia. Pain referring along the same fascial sector or sequence marked the breakdown in the harmonious functioning of what he called the *myofascial unit*. While Stecco speaks Italian and French, his English is not fluent. The opportunity of discussing his ideas within this Symposium setting would have been quite restricted but his enthusiasm and tenaciousness could not have been doubted.

Stecco's second book (Figure I.4), published in 1990, was entitled '*Il dolore e le sequenze neuro-mio-fasciali*' (in English: '*Pain and the neuro-myo-fascial sequences*'). It included an evaluation process for fascial dysfunction, a treatment methodology, and a procedure of post-treatment reassessment, and it proposed possible research avenues into internal or visceral dysfunctions. A poster presented at the Second World Congress on Myofascial Pain held in 1992 in Copenhagen, comparing trigger points and Maigne's areas

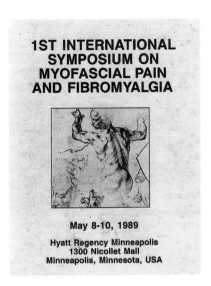

Figure I.3

Flyer of the First International Symposium on Myofascial Pain and Fibromyalgia, Minneapolis (USA), 1989. Courtesy of Luigi Stecco

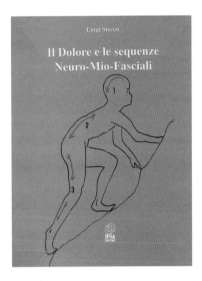

Figure I.4

Cover of the second Italian-language book concerning the human fascial system published by Luigi Stecco in 1990. Courtesy of Luigi Stecco

with Stecco's own fascial points, must have represented yet another challenge for his communication skills! In the meantime, Stecco published a few clinical research articles in a French journal (*Annales de Kinésithérapie*) and an Italian physiotherapy journal (*La Riabilitazione*), presenting the idea that, in rehabilitation, it was important to consider entire movement patterns rather than single muscle activity, and introducing the concept of *myofascial units* and *myofascial sequences* to provide a better understanding of the role of fascia within the musculoskeletal system.

In 1995, Stecco began teaching his manual method, initially called 'Neuroconnective Manipulation.' Courses have continued to be popular throughout Italy ever since, but Stecco's proposals did not become widely accessible internationally until 2004, when the first English edition of *Fascial Manipulation for Musculoskeletal Pain* (Stecco L. 2004) was published. About that time, the name Fascial Manipulation® was officially adopted for the method. More recently it has been modified to Fascial Manipulation®–Stecco® method.

In 2007, the First International Fascial Research Congress held at the Harvard Medical School Conference Center in Boston (USA) represented a first-time showcase opportunity to present both an introduction to Luigi Stecco's method and the high quality fascial anatomy research that was being conducted by his daughter, Carla Stecco. (Professor Carla Stecco, an orthopedic surgeon and professor of anatomy, and her brother, Dr Antonio Stecco, specialist in physical medicine and rehabilitation, have since published over 100 indexed articles that examine the anatomy, histology, and physiology of fascia, as well as numerous clinical research papers.) Meanwhile, courses had also started in Spain, South America, and Poland.

In 2008, the founding of the Fascial Manipulation Association furnished an initial organizational framework for the diffusion of the method, followed by the formation of the Fascial Manipulation Institute, directed by the Stecco family since 2016.

Shortly after the publication of an English edition of *Fascial Manipulation for Musculoskeletal Dysfunctions: Practical Part* (Stecco L. & Stecco C. 2009), a 1-day introductory workshop to FM, was presented for the first time at the Second International Fascia Research Congress held in Amsterdam. This workshop was attended by professionals from different disciplines and led to the first English language course of FM being held in Italy in June 2010. Manual therapists from the USA, Canada, Denmark, and a number of other countries attended this course and it became a catalyst for spreading the method. Several contributors to this book attended that first course.

By this stage, FM for musculoskeletal dysfunctions was well-defined and, while improvements in the method continue to be introduced, the basic principles have remained unaltered.

Luigi Stecco can be described as a methodical person with an innate curiosity. Over the last 45 years, he has studied and written in the morning and treated patients in the afternoon. This untiring dedication has led to a further development, *Fascial Manipulation® for Internal Dysfunctions* (FMID). In his 1990 book, Stecco had already spoken of internal dysfunctions connected with three autonomic systems that correspond to the internal pathways of the principal meridians. Further inspired by the works of Michel Coquillat (1995), when the first Italian editions of Jean-Pierre Barral's work were published (Barral & Mercier 1998) he also studied these extensively, gathering information but still maintaining his own individual view.

Luigi Stecco first presented his ideas regarding internal organs, their supportive fasciae, and their interaction with the autonomic nervous system (ANS) in 2002. Since then, an entire methodology has been developed, incorporating treatment for internal apparatus dysfunctions as well as system dysfunctions involving the superficial fascia. Pertinent theoretical and practical texts (Stecco L. & Stecco C. 2014; Stecco L. & Stecco A. 2016) have introduced these concepts to an international audience, and courses addressing this approach are presently held regularly in Italy and elsewhere. In 2016, Luigi Stecco published an atlas of the physiology of fascia (Stecco L. 2016) that presents a detailed description of the normal physiology of fascia together with numerous functional applications.

Luigi Stecco rarely travels outside of Italy, preferring to assign the task of spreading his ideas to his son, Dr Antonio Stecco, who travels extensively, teaching, lecturing at international conferences, and collaborating with numerous research projects throughout the world. International lectures, courses, and dissection workshops are also held by Professor Carla Stecco, who is the author of an unprecedented atlas of human fascial anatomy (Stecco C. 2015). Luigi Stecco's books have now been translated into 11 different languages and a growing team of qualified instructors teaches FM courses around the world.

The models applied in the Fascial Manipulation®–Stecco® method

Initially focusing on the relationship between muscular fascia and the musculoskeletal system, Stecco first integrated his studies about fascia with his clinical experience to develop a biomechanical model that relates fascial dysfunction to movement limitation, weakness, and pain distribution. He later developed a second model for application to internal dysfunctions involving visceral fasciae and their interrelationships with muscular fasciae. In effect, his life's work has been directed towards simplifying the very complex interrelationship that exists between fascia, muscle, bone, internal apparatus, and systems. Here the two models are presented briefly and the assessment process used by therapists is discussed. Readers are invited to consult the Stecco texts for a complete explanation of the theoretical background and its practical applications.

Stecco's model for musculoskeletal dysfunctions

This model presents a paradigmatic change in the analysis of dysfunctions by considering the fascia as an active component of the musculoskeletal system. As movement is a continuous flux of motor units that activates parts of muscles according to the degree of joint movement, direction, and force required, Stecco promptly discarded individual muscles as functional units. He turned to motor units as the baseline for muscular function, thereby overcoming the paradox of single muscles that perform multiple functions. Motor units activate their relative muscle fibers in an all-or-nothing manner and, curiously, these fibers are not always adjacent to one another and can even be located in different muscles.

Stecco realized that the 'fascial skeleton' within muscular tissue could act as the uniting element for these non-adjacent muscle fibers. He proposed that the musculoskeletal system could be interpreted in terms of *myofascial units* (mf unit). (Please note that this model introduces a series of new terms and associated abbreviations that can initially present a challenge, justifiable by the paradigmatic vision of the musculoskeletal system that it depicts. These terms are highlighted here in *italics* and a Glossary is supplied (see pp. ix–x)).

Each mf unit is composed of:

- motor units that innervate monoarticular and biarticular muscle fibers
- the joint these muscle fibers move in one direction on one plane
- the nerve components involved in this movement
- the deep fascia and its derivatives (epimysium, perimysium, and endomysium), which unite the above components.

One example is the mf unit for elbow extension: the joint component is the elbow; the fascia of the posterior upper limb forms the fascial component; and the muscular component is formed by motor units that activate fibers of the medial and lateral heads of triceps (monoarticular) and the long head of triceps (biarticular) to bring about elbow extension (Figure I.5). This same combination of basic components can be found in all mf units; therefore, they can be considered as the 'building blocks' of the myofascial system.

Stecco divided the body into 14 functional segments (Figure I.6) composed of parts of muscles, one or more

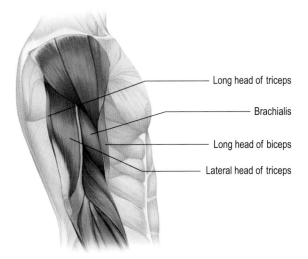

Long head of triceps

Brachialis

Long head of biceps

Lateral head of triceps

Figure I.5

The myofascial unit for elbow extension consists of the elbow, the fascia of the posterior upper limb and the motor units that activate fibers of the medial and lateral heads of triceps (monoarticular fibers) and the long head of triceps (biarticular fibers)

related joints, and their fascial surround. Latin names distinguish these segments from mere joints (Stecco L. 2004).

Six mf units regulate the movement of each body segment on the three spatial planes (sagittal, horizontal, and frontal), providing multiple vectors that act on each segment and guaranteeing that each mf unit has control over movement in one direction. The monoarticular fibers provide strength and stability during movement, while the biarticular fibers transmit tension between adjoining segments, ensuring coordinated movement. By linking unidirectional mf units, the biarticular component contributes to the formation of *myofascial sequences*. A single myofascial sequence is said to synchronize the movement of body segments in one direction on one plane, while sequences on the same spatial plane can be considered as reciprocal antagonists.

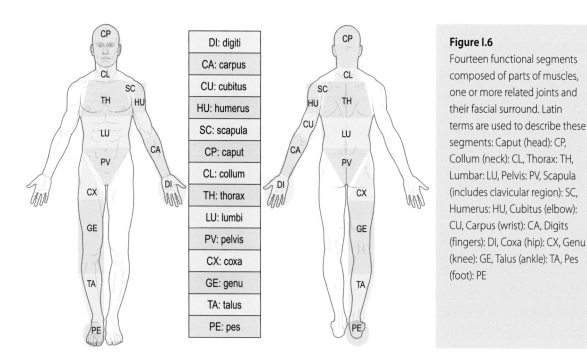

DI: digiti
CA: carpus
CU: cubitus
HU: humerus
SC: scapula
CP: caput
CL: collum
TH: thorax
LU: lumbi
PV: pelvis
CX: coxa
GE: genu
TA: talus
PE: pes

Figure I.6

Fourteen functional segments composed of parts of muscles, one or more related joints and their fascial surround. Latin terms are used to describe these segments: Caput (head): CP, Collum (neck): CL, Thorax: TH, Lumbar: LU, Pelvis: PV, Scapula (includes clavicular region): SC, Humerus: HU, Cubitus (elbow): CU, Carpus (wrist): CA, Digits (fingers): DI, Coxa (hip): CX, Genu (knee): GE, Talus (ankle): TA, Pes (foot): PE

Each mf unit has a:

- *center of coordination* (CC), which is a small area mostly located over the epimysium of the monoarticular component, where the forces involved in muscle fiber contraction converge. Myofascial tension within an mf unit can converge at a CC because part of the epimysial fascia slides freely over the underlying muscle fibers and part of the deep fascia, which connects with the epimysial fascia, is anchored to the bone via intermuscular septa

- *center of perception* (CP), which is situated in a circumscribed area over the joint capsule, tendons and ligaments that are tensioned when the muscle fibers of a mf unit contract. The CP is where movement resulting from mf unit activity is perceived.

The continuity of endomysium (which surrounds each muscle fiber) with perimysium (surrounding muscle fiber groups) and epimysium (surrounding each muscle and continuing with deep fascia) could permit harmonious synchronization of all these tensional forces during movement. Theoretically, if gliding between intrafascial collagen fibers in the area of the CC is impeded, then pain can be felt in the area of the CP.

As movements are commonly multidirectional, other small areas of deep fascia, called *centers of fusion* (CF), have been identified. CFs are said to monitor movements in intermediate directions between two planes, as well as movements of adjacent segments in different directions. CFs are located principally over retinacula and around joints and combinations of CFs are linked either by longitudinal collagen fibers to form myofascial diagonals or via obliquely orientated collagen fibers to form myofascial spirals.

Clinically, Stecco noted that the fascia in these intersecting points of tension (CCs and CFs) is commonly subject to palpable changes called '*densification*' (Figure I.7), which differs from fascial 'fibrosis' (Pavan et al. 2014). He observed that by applying deep friction to these small densified areas, pain at the CPs reduces significantly and normal movement can be rapidly restored.

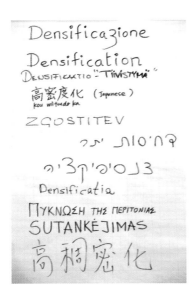

Figure I.7
Densification translated into different languages by an international group of participants during a course in 2012

Anatomical findings and possible physiological mechanisms

Studies led by Professor Carla Stecco have demonstrated that deep fascia consists of multilayered collagen fiber bundles interspersed with elastic fibers and each layer is separated from the next by loose connective tissue, which allows for interlayer sliding. Furthermore, each adjacent collagen fiber layer is aligned in a different direction creating an aponeurotic type structure. The angle between the fibers of adjacent layers in both crural fascia and thoracolumbar fascia is approximately 80° (Benetazzo et al. 2011). As a whole, this type of structure permits a certain degree of stretch plus the capacity to recoil and ensures that fascia's response to loading varies according to the direction (Stecco C. et al. 2009).

While biarticular muscular fibers can clearly connect two segments together, in his attentive reading of anatomy texts Luigi Stecco noted that the majority of muscles also have fibers that insert directly onto deep fascia, and that

deep fascia in one segment connects with deep fascia in the adjacent segment, yet no functional reason had ever been proposed for these well-documented connections. Anatomical dissections have since demonstrated that important myofascial connections are consistently present between the various body segments (Stecco C. et al. 2008; Stecco A. et al. 2009), confirming the anatomical continuity between the deep fascia of adjacent segments and, together with the biarticular muscular fibers, providing the anatomical substratum of myofascial sequences.

Innervation of the fascia was a key element in determining its potential role in myofascial pain. While Luigi Stecco initially hypothesized that fascia was innervated tissue, histological studies have since demonstrated that deep fascia is, indeed, well innervated with free nerve endings, as well as some Pacini and Ruffini corpuscles (Stecco C. et al. 2006, 2008; Tesarz et al. 2011).

Furthermore, important interactions occur between muscle spindle activity and fasciae via the connective tissue capsule of the muscle spindle (Stecco L. 2016). Muscle spindles are situated in parallel to muscle fibers, immersed in endomysium, which permits sliding, and their capsule is attached to the perimysium, which adapts to the stretch generated from contraction of the muscle spindles' intrafusal fibers. Stecco proposes that this continuity ensures that, via the gamma-alpha circuit, this stretch activates the motor units innervating those extrafusal fibers that are involved in a specific direction of movement.

Therefore, Stecco hypothesizes that abnormal tensioning within the fascial skeleton has the potential to alter muscle spindle firing, resulting in incomplete recruitment of muscle fibers and subsequent malalignment of joint movement, indicating a role for fasciae in peripheral motor coordination.

Stecco's model for internal dysfunctions

Luigi Stecco's model for the internal fasciae provides a new vision of the role of these fasciae in the physiology and pathology of internal organs and their interactions with the musculoskeletal system, superficial fascia, and ANS. This model has led to the development of FMID.

Stecco divides internal fasciae into two types: (1) *investing fasciae* that adhere to the viscera, vessels, and glands and are closely related to the organ walls; (2) *insertional fasciae* that form specific compartments, providing vital spaces to isolate organs from the external environment and from other organs (Stecco C. et al. 2017). However, insertional fasciae also connect different organs in longitudinal and transverse directions and provide attachments to the trunk wall and muscular fasciae at specific points via mesenteries and internal ligaments.

Based on the premise that elasticity and physiological tensioning of internal fasciae is a fundamental element for correct internal organ peristalsis, patency of internal spaces, and the motility and mobility of the organs contained within these spaces, the FMID approach focuses on small, rigid areas on the trunk wall that can potentially interfere with internal fasciae tension and, thereby, influence autonomic function. Autonomic intramural plexuses implanted within investing fasciae are very sensitive to changes in organ volume and they transmit information to the extramural ganglia, which are embedded in insertional fasciae. Insertional fasciae are also innervated by somatic nerves and therefore can transmit nociceptive signals.

Once again, palpation is used to identify rigid points. In reference to the FMID model, associated points on the trunk wall are then treated manually until physiological elasticity is restored. Treatment may be completed with affiliated *pivot points* located in the shoulder and pelvic girdles and *distal tensor points* located in the ankles, feet, wrists, and hands. The points used in FMID treatments are predominately the same as those used in musculoskeletal treatments but the association of points and the modality and logic of treatment differs.

L. Stecco fully acknowledges Jean-Pierre Barral's extensive work on visceral manipulation and has taken inspiration from this author. (The fact that J.-P. Barral wrote the preface to the first edition of L. Stecco's internal dysfunction text implies that the recognition is mutual.) However, the FMID approach does not act directly on the fascia of the organs but on the fascia of

their 'container,' namely the trunk wall. Hence, FMID can be considered an indirect approach that influences internal organs and systems by acting on key areas related to internal fasciae. This is somewhat similar to acupuncture, which addresses numerous internal dysfunctions by inserting needles into the superficial and deep fasciae of the trunk wall without directly piercing the fasciae of internal organs.

The FMID approach is particularly indicated when medical investigations have excluded any internal pathologies. Signs of internal dysfunction include abnormal sensations such as abdominal swelling, irregular bowel movements, gastroesophageal reflux, globus pharyngeus, and diffuse, poorly localized pain.

A distinction is made between disturbances that are localized in one segment, or in an entire apparatus, or involving a system.

Internal dysfunctions localized in one segment

Similar to his interpretation of the musculoskeletal system, with FMID Stecco introduces the concept of *organ-fascial units* (o-f units) and their dependency on normal autonomic intramural and extramural ganglia activity for correct peristalsis. Engineering principles related to *tensile structures* are applied for single segment disturbances that may imitate an internal organ disorder. The FMID model considers the external fasciae of the trunk wall as being similar to tensile structures that form cavities within the trunk without taking mechanical leverage on the organs within. At the same time, the trunk wall receives insertions from mesenteries and internal ligaments (*insertional fasciae*), and the body's tensile structures must allow for adaptation to external stress as well as guaranteeing an adequate response to the motor needs of the musculoskeletal system.

Internal dysfunctions related to apparatus-fascial sequences

Stecco defines an apparatus as being formed by individual organs that collaborate together for a single function and are connected together by insertional fasciae. Dysfunctions within an apparatus can affect several o-f units and, owing to transverse connections via the insertional fasciae, can potentially influence other apparatus.

FMID considers six apparatus within the trunk:

- respiratory (includes the larynx in the neck and the lungs in the thorax)
- digestive (includes the lumbar (stomach) and pelvic (intestine) regions)
- circulatory (includes the heart and the blood vessels)
- urinary (includes the kidney, urinary bladder, retroperitoneal vessels, urethra)
- endocrine (includes endocrine glands such as the pineal, hypophysis, thyroid, parathyroid, pericardium, liver, pancreas, adrenals, ovaries and prostate)
- hematopoietic (includes bone marrow, liver, thymus, spleen and lymph nodes that all produce cellular components of blood)

and three receptor apparatus in the head cavities:

- photoreceptor (related to sight and stereopsis)
- mechanoreceptor (related to hearing and statokinetics)
- chemoreceptor (related to olfaction and taste).

The activity of an apparatus is dependent on the correct tautness of investing and insertional fasciae, which can be altered by abnormal tension along so-called *catenaries* in the trunk and head, as well as distal tensors in the limbs.

Apparatus are also connected in series by longitudinal internal fascial sequences to form *apparatus-fascial sequences* (a-f sequences) that synchronize the activity of the extramural enteric plexuses in order to coordinate the various o-f units that form each a-f sequence.

Internal dysfunctions within systems

Within the FMID concept, a system is considered to be the union of parts that are organized in a similar manner and which extend throughout the entire body.

Stecco identifies three systems:

1. cutaneous-thermoregulatory
2. lymphatic-immune
3. adipose-metabolic.

To each system he assigns an external component, connected with the hypodermis, which includes the superficial fascia, as well as an internal component.

Systems do not function via stretch because they are connected with the superficial fascia, which is a more elastic layer. Instead, they communicate with the prevertebral and paravertebral ganglia via autonomic afferents and efferents, and their role is to maintain homeostasis between the body's internal functions and any external perturbations by triggering reactions to stress.

There is also a fourth system, the psychogenic system, related to the emotional components that can affect a person. Psychogenic dysfunctions can be psycho-somatic or somato-psychic and, depending on which tissue is altered, treatment is directed at either the superficial or the muscular fascia.

For systemic dysfunctions, distinct manual approaches are proposed for the lymphatic system, for the mobilization of the adipose system, and for freeing peripheral nerves from any localized deposits of densified fascial tissue.

The assessment process

The assessment process used in FM respects the indications given for a scientific approach, which includes observation, measurement, and the formulation, testing, and modification of a hypothesis. All practitioners who have completed basic training are well-informed about the models used in FM and the relevant contraindications. For example, feverish states and recent thrombosis or skin lesions in the area of treatment are contraindications to applying this method.

Therapists applying the FM method use a specific assessment chart (Figure I.8) for the analysis of fascial dysfunction. This chart is compiled using standardized

N°	Segments	Locat	Side	Durat (acu-1)	T/?	VRS (n-M)	Rec/con	Painful Movements:	
Si Pa									
Pa Conc									Name:
Extremit.	CP								
	DI								Surname:
	PE								
Pa Prev								Investigations:	Date of birth
								Medications:	
Surgery								Internal dysf.:	Occupation:
Trauma Fracture								Posture:	Sports:

HYP.	A	D	(lt) SAGITTAL (rt)		(lt an) FRONTAL (rt)		(lt) HORIZONTAL (rt)		Others MoVe:							
	SEGM.		ANTE	RETRO	MEDIO	LATERO	INTRA	EXTRA								
M O V E									AN-ME		RE-LA		RE-ME		AN-LA	
									lt	rt	lt	rt	lt	rt	lt	rt
P A V E																

		Outcomes	Now	
			2° treat	

Figure I.8

An example of the method-specific assessment chart used during the assessment process and clinical reasoning applied in FM.
SiPa = site of pain; Pa Conc = concomitant pain; PaPrev = previous pain; HYP = hypothesis

abbreviations and it involves a subjective and an objective examination.

Subjective assessment

The subjective examination, or patient interview, includes information regarding:

- age, occupation, and sports

- location of symptoms, duration, verbal rating scale (VRS), quality of pain/disturbance, and any known

painful movement(s) related to the main dysfunction and to any concomitant dysfunctions

- previous musculoskeletal dysfunctions of note that are currently asymptomatic

- symptoms and signs in the extremities, previous surgery or fractures, visceral dysfunctions, and general health.

To formulate a hypothesis, particular attention is given to the chronology of events regarding the primary cause, or causes, of dysfunction. The subjective examination may indicate a hypothesis for a primarily musculoskeletal dysfunction or a predominately internal dysfunction, which then directs the therapist to the appropriate model to apply in the objective assessment and treatment.

Objective assessment and treatment procedure for musculoskeletal dysfunctions

If the hypothesis indicates a primary musculoskeletal dysfunction, then the spread of tensional compensations from one body segment to another is closely considered. Two or three potentially dysfunctional body segments are selected for the objective examination, which initially consists of standardized movement tests. The aim of these movement tests is to examine the quality of movement of a segment on the three spatial planes in terms of range, strength, and pain.

The next step is a comparative palpation of CCs and CFs around selected segments. The aim of comparative palpation is to identify a pattern of densified areas within the deep muscular fascia of these key areas. Once the therapist identifies a pattern within a 'fascial structure' (considered to be a plane, a myofascial diagonal, or a myofascial spiral), then treatment focuses on that structure during a session. Therapists use deep friction over the densified areas within that structure, keeping in mind either tensional balance on a plane or the relationship between CFs in adjacent segments, whether it be along a myofascial diagonal or a myofascial spiral.

Given the implications of deep fascia in musculoskeletal dysfunction and myofascial pain (Stecco A. et al. 2016), the aim of treatment is to modify the extracellular matrix of the intrafascial loose connective tissue layers by inducing chain reactions in the hyaluronan component of these layers, transforming the tissue's state from gel to sol. Deep tangential oscillating friction is suggested to be the preferable manual approach to affect hyaluronan flow around fascia (Roman et al. 2013).

Any faulty movements identified earlier in the objective assessment, by means of the standardized movement tests, are used as an immediate post-treatment evaluation of treatment efficacy.

Objective assessment and treatment procedure for internal dysfunctions

If the hypothesis indicates an internal dysfunction as the primary source of reported disturbances, then therapists refer to Stecco's biomechanical model for internal dysfunctions (FMID). In FMID, movement tests are also performed but greater emphasis is placed on comparative palpation of tensile structures, catenaries, and superficial fascia quadrants in reference to the divisions into organ-fascial units (o-f units), apparatus-fascial sequences (a-f sequences), and systems. With o-f unit and a-f sequence dysfunctions, therapists identify a pattern of altered CCs and CFs (the same points also used in musculoskeletal dysfunctions) that are potentially interfering with internal organ motility and the interaction between the components of an apparatus. These points are located principally on the trunk wall, head, shoulder girdle, and pelvic girdle, but also in the distal segments of the extremities. With system dysfunctions, quadrants of superficial fascia are targeted in order to improve lymphatic drainage, adipose metabolism, or peripheral nerve entrapments.

Importance of clinical expertise in the evidence-based practice model

Evidenced-based practice (EBP), an offspring of evidence-based medicine (EBM), is vitally important in clinical work. However, it is often overlooked that clinical experience and expertise is an important aspect of the original EBM/EBP concept. In effect, the triad of EBM is based on clinical expertise, patient values and preferences, and the best available research, with each aspect having equal validity (Figure I.9).

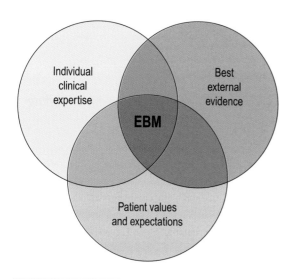

Figure I.9

The evidence-based medicine triad

Not all practitioners are in a position to carry out clinical research studies themselves. Nevertheless, they are able to discern patients' needs and preferences. The soundest decisions are made with the patient and are not necessarily taken from journals and books (Herbert et al. 2001). In the best models of EBP, evidence about the effects of therapy (or accuracy of diagnostic tests or prognoses) informs but does not dominate clinical decision-making. Therapists necessarily draw on their clinical experience to apply the results of research in the care of individual patients.

Emphasis is generally placed on published research as the most important aspect of EBP but, as D. L. Sackett (Sackett et al. 1996), one of the primary promoters of the EBM model in the 1990s, states: 'External clinical evidence can inform, but can never replace, individual clinical expertise, and it is this expertise that decides whether the external evidence applies to the individual patient at all and, if so, how it should be integrated into a clinical decision.'

Integrating a new model into one's work is a challenge for established professionals, yet it is a necessary part of a clinician's obligation to their patients to provide them with the best available treatment. Randomized trials or systematic reviews of randomized trials are considered paramount evidence but what happens if a professional learns of new methods that have yet to be fully investigated but provide consistent results when they are applied clinically? Responsible practitioners necessarily work within a no-harm framework but new models can provide new insights.

In anatomy, fascia is still a lesser known tissue, even though it has always been there. While muscular and visceral fasciae are gaining attention in areas of anatomy, physiology, and manual therapies, the amount of published qualitative research regarding clinical evidence is still relatively limited. The case reports in this book represent testimonials of manual therapy professionals regarding their experiences with two models that (1) place muscular fascia in an active role within the musculoskeletal system and (2) address the interrelationships of visceral and superficial fasciae with the musculoskeletal system, internal organs and apparatus, and the homeostatic systems.

References

Barral J-P and Mercier P (1998) Manipolazione viscerale 1. Milan: Castello Editore.

Benetazzo L, Bizzego A, De Caro R, Frigo G, Guidolin D and Stecco C (2011) 3D reconstruction of the crural and thoracolumbar fasciae. Surgical and Radiologic Anatomy 33 (10) 855–62. doi: 10.1007/s00276-010-0757-7.

Coquillat M (1995) L'osteopatia viscerale. Rome: Marrapese.

Herbert RD, Sherrington C, Maher C and Moseley AM (2001) Evidence-based practice: Imperfect but necessary. Physiotherapy Theory and Practice 17 (3) 201–11. doi:10.1080/095939801317077650

Pavan PG, Stecco A, Stern R and Stecco C (2014) Painful connections: Densification versus fibrosis of fascia. Current Pain and Headache Reports 18 (8) 441. doi: 10.1007/s11916-014-0441-4.

Roman M, Chaudhry H, Bukiet B, Stecco A and Findley TW (2013) Mathematical analysis of the flow of hyaluronic acid around fascia during manual therapy motions. Journal of the American Osteopathic Association 113 (8) 600–10. doi: 10.7556/jaoa.2013.021.

Sackett DL, Rosenberg WMC, Muir Gray JA, Haynes RB and Scott Richardson W (1996)

Evidence based medicine: What it is and what it isn't. BMJ 312 71–2.

Stecco A, Macchi V, Stecco C, Porzionato A, Ann Day J, Delmas V and De Caro R (2009) Anatomical study of myofascial continuity in the anterior region of the upper limb. Journal of Bodywork and Movement Therapies 13 (1) 53–62.

Stecco A, Stern R, Fantoni I, De Caro R and Stecco C (2016) Fascial disorders: Implications for treatment. PM & R 8 (2) 161–8. doi: 10.1016/j.pmrj.2015.06.006.

Stecco C (2015) Functional atlas of the human fascial system. Edinburgh: Churchill Livingstone, Elsevier.

Stecco C, Porzionato A, Macchi V, Tiengo C, Parenti A, Aldegheri R, Delmas V and De Caro R (2006) A histological study of the deep fascia of the upper limb. Italian Journal of Anatomy and Embryology 111 (2) 105–10.

Stecco C, Porzionato A, Lancerotto L, Stecco A, Macchi V, Day JA and De Caro R (2008) Histological study of the deep fasciae of the limbs. Journal of Bodywork and Movement Therapies 12 (3) 225–30.

Stecco C, Pavan PG, Porzionato A, Macchi V, Lancerotto L, Carniel EL, Natali AN and De Caro R (2009) Mechanics of crural fascia:

From anatomy to constitutive modelling. Surgical and Radiologic Anatomy 31 523–9.

Stecco C, Sfriso MM, Porzionato A, Rambaldo A, Albertin G, Macchi V and De Caro R (2017) Microscopic anatomy of the visceral fasciae. Journal of Anatomy 231 (1) 121–8.

Stecco L (1987) Sequenze neuro-mio-fasciali e meridiani agopunturei. Arzignano: Molin.

Stecco L (1990) Il dolore e le sequenze neuro-mio-fasciali. Palermo: Nuova IPSA.

Stecco L (2004) Fascial manipulation for musculoskeletal pain. Padua: Piccin.

Stecco L (2016) Atlas of physiology of the muscular fascia. Padua: Piccin.

Stecco L and Stecco A (2016) Fascial manipulation for internal dysfunctions: Practical part. Padua: Piccin.

Stecco L and Stecco C (2009) Fascial manipulation: Practical part. Padua: Piccin.

Stecco L and Stecco C (2014) Fascial manipulation for internal dysfunctions. Padua: Piccin.

Tesarz J, Hoheisel U, Wiedenhöfer B and Mense S (2011) Sensory innervation of the thoracolumbar fascia in rats and humans. Neuroscience 194 302–8.

Section 1
Musculoskeletal dysfunctions

This section contains five chapters dealing with the treatment of musculoskeletal dysfunctions. According to Luigi Stecco, these types of dysfunction are generally caused by densification of the deep fascia, which can be divided into aponeurotic and epimysial-type fasciae. Stecco hypothesizes that alteration of these fasciae affects muscle spindle and Golgi tendon organ activity, with repercussions on peripheral motor coordination that lead to tensional compensations and compensatory movement strategies. Myofascial and joint pain are said to develop when tensional compensations are no longer functionally effective. In these five chapters, the authors refer to Stecco's biomechanical model for musculoskeletal dysfunctions to trace back to the origin of the tensional compensations that have developed in each individual case.

Treatment of low back pain in a female athlete

Mirco Branchini, Italy

EDITOR'S COMMENT

The author of this chapter attended Luigi Stecco's first course in Bologna, Italy, in 1995. This course, titled Neuroconnective Manipulation, developed over time to become Fascial Manipulation and, more recently, the Fascial Manipulation®–Stecco® (FM) method. The case report presented here details the resolution of low back pain in a semi-professional volleyball player after a single session of FM. Movement tests for the myofascial sequences are used to analyze faulty movement and instability. These tests differ from movement tests for individual segments as they involve a series of isometric loads applied in the six directions of movement on the three spatial planes (see the Glossary entry: Directions of movement), allowing therapists to test all the trunk segments and/or limbs simultaneously. The author describes how the outcome of these movement tests influenced his clinical reasoning process and how aspects were then confirmed or modified by palpation verification, culminating in the choice of specific fascial points for the treatment. The final discussion highlights key aspects related to the biomechanical model of the fascial system, as proposed by Stecco, that physiotherapists should consider when applying this method.

Author's background

I graduated as a physiotherapist from the USL n.28 School of Physiotherapy, Bologna, Italy, in 1992, and in 2006 I obtained a master's degree from the University of Florence. I have always worked in public health care structures (hospitals and health centers), treating a wide variety of acute and chronic disorders in adults, including areas of orthopedics, rheumatology, and neurology. As part of my postgraduate education I have completed courses in Global Postural Re-

education (1992), McKenzie (1997), Bobath (2000) and, of course, the Fascial Manipulation®–Stecco® (FM) method. I attended Luigi Stecco's very first course in Italy in 1995, followed by many other courses over the years. Since 1997, I have been a member of the physiotherapy degree course faculty at the University of Bologna, where I teach a number of subjects, including rehabilitation of the peripheral nervous system and an elective course called 'Introduction to Fascial Manipulation®–Stecco® method'. In 2007 I took on the position of Didactic Coordinator for this degree course.

Experience with Fascial Manipulation®–Stecco® method

When I attended Luigi Stecco's first course in 1995 I immediately realized that this concept was tailor-made for me. There are three features I really like about FM. The first is the biomechanical model, because it considers fascia and its relationship with muscle fibers, which explains functional anatomy easily and the reason why all movement should be interpreted in terms of myofascial units, the basic units of our movement system, rather than muscles. Functional anatomy as proposed by Stecco explains how the body-wide myofascial system works to ensure stability and tensional balance throughout the body.

Secondly, I like how patients are assessed with the FM procedure. As the myofascial system is an entire complex structure, all items in the initial anamnesis, or patient history, refer to a unique tensional imbalance. Physiotherapists can then assess this imbalance objectively by using movement verifications, including simple functional tests, and palpatory verifications that involve examination of myofascial tissues with fingers and knuckles. Combining the hypothesis formulated from the data collected during anamnesis with the objective evaluation, the physiotherapist elaborates a personalized treatment plan for each individual.

The third aspect I really love about FM is the manual sensation that I have when I am applying deep friction

CHAPTER 1

to fascial tissue. It is amazing to perceive how easy it is to modify tissue during treatment and how pain improves as tissue planes glide better.

Working with students at the university I have had the opportunity of performing numerous clinical trials concerning FM. It was not surprising for me to discover how straightforward it was for these university students to learn the FM method and how they were able to treat all the subjects enrolled in these trials with excellent results.

In my own clinical practice, I use FM as my first approach, especially to assess the presenting impairment. This deductive and logical way to study pain and limitation in range of movement (ROM) enables me to analyze the patient's entire history in order to get to the cause of the dysfunction.

Although FM is almost always effective, I never forget that a physiotherapist may need to use other techniques to complete the results. After an FM treatment, I have found that muscular or joint techniques are easier to perform in the following sessions, allowing for an integrated approach. Nevertheless, despite the fact that this type of treatment is initially a little painful, once patients know that FM enables them to move better because it can reduce pain on movement almost immediately, they will often ask for treatment of the densified points that have been found.

CASE REPORT

Treatment of low back pain in a female athlete

Introduction

E. is a 26-year-old semi-professional volleyball player who presented with right-sided posterolateral lumbar pain. The pain had been present for about 4 months and it had started without a particular cause, although there was a correlation between pain onset and the beginning of the training season. Unable to continue playing due to this pain, E. was forced to interrupt her athletic training for

3 weeks. During that time, she had physiotherapy treatment and some reconditioning activities. The pain subsided but was not entirely resolved and it recurred with greater intensity when full agonistic training was resumed.

When first assessed, E. was unable to practice sport and the pain also limited some daily activities, such as prolonged standing, standing up from an armchair, and sleeping on one side, in particular, on the right side. When the pain was more pronounced it also referred down the posterolateral part of her right leg, to halfway down her thigh. At those peak times, E. reported that pain was 8/10 on a visual analog scale (VAS). One month prior to assessment, magnetic resonance imaging (MRI) of the lumbar region had highlighted right-sided paramedian disc protrusions at the L3–4 and L4–5 levels, a minor scoliosis of the lumbar region, convex on the right-side, and flattening of the lumbar lordosis. E. was taking painkillers for the pain. After 7–8 days of ibuprofen without significant results, her club's doctor had suggested that she begin cortisone, but she decided to wait for the results of our treatment before taking it and was continuing postural exercises under the supervision of a physiotherapist.

The patient's previous history included several traumas to the fingers in both hands, fortunately fairly minor, and a bimalleolar compound fracture to her left ankle that had occurred approximately 10 months previously, during a game of volleyball. The fracture had not required surgery but her ankle was in a cast for 30 days. She had also had an appendectomy 8 years previously. There were no other musculoskeletal symptoms and when questioned about internal dysfunctions, she reported that bowel movements were regular and a recent gynecological examination had not detected any anomalies.

Hypothesis

Based on the above information, clinical reasoning was immediately directed towards a soft tissue problem because:

- no lumbar trauma was reported prior to the onset of the presenting problem

- it was unlikely that the disc protrusions could be the cause of a symptom that refers along the lower limb and, even more so, their location could not justify a posterolateral distribution of pain

- there were no other indications for an involvement of joints in the painful segment

- internal dysfunctions were not present

- previous physiotherapy focused on postural control and core stability exercises had given only temporary relief.

Therefore, having excluded red and yellow flags, the formulation of a hypothesis was the next step. It involved, as always, consideration of the chronology of the two known traumatic events that had occurred prior to the onset of E.'s presenting symptoms: the bimalleolar ankle fracture and the appendectomy surgery. Both events could be related to the presenting problem because:

- the surgery was located in the proximity of the currently painful body segment

- most activities that provoked the pain involved use of the lower limbs, therefore, the involvement of the left ankle was more than probable.

Hence, a treatment using the FM method was deemed appropriate and all of the segments mentioned in the anamnesis were taken into consideration.

Methodology

Movement verification (MoVe)

For the movement verification (MoVe), tests for the myofascial sequences were used (Stecco L. & Stecco A. 2017). These tests are different from the movement tests for individual segments. They allow the therapist to test all the trunk segments and/or the limbs simultaneously. A series of isometric loads is applied, for example, to the head when testing the trunk, in the six directions of movement on the three spatial planes (sagittal, frontal, and horizontal). The subject has to maintain stability in all segments simultaneously, as the therapist applies a static force (Figure 1.1). The test is considered to be

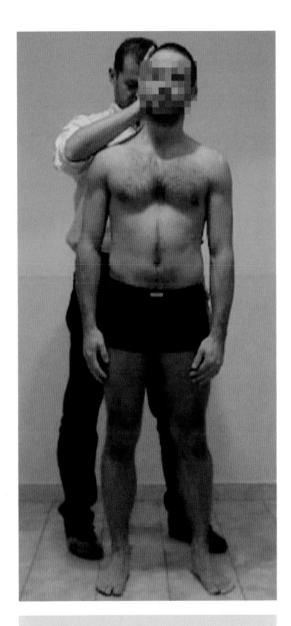

Figure 1.1

Test of the sequences in standing. In this photograph the physiotherapist applies a force to the right side of the patient's head, in the temporoparietal region, in order to stimulate recruitment of the lateral myofascial units, or lateromotion sequence, of the trunk on the same side. In addition, the resistance of the subject should also involve a counteraction of the left lower limb on the ground

CHAPTER 1

positive if the subject is either unable to maintain stability in one or more segments or if their pain is reproduced. In this particular case, the possibility to apply these tests in standing or sitting (Figure 1.2) allowed the therapist to verify whether the previous left ankle fracture was a relevant factor in E.'s stability. In effect, if the test was found to be more significant in standing as opposed to sitting, then there would be a strong indication that the ankle segment (talus: ta) should be included in the treatment. (For an explanation of method-specific terminology for directions of movement consult the Glossary entry: Directions of movement.)

The test of the sequences in standing highlighted:

- frontal plane: isometric holding of the lateromotion sequence on the right caused referred pain along the right lower limb together with instability of the left lower limb, which should normally counteract the contralateral force applied by the therapist; isometric holding in a lateral direction on the left was negative

- sagittal plane: isometric holding applied from posterior to anterior to test the sequence of retromotion caused pain in the right lumbar region; isometric holding, applied from anterior to posterior to test the antemotion sequence, evidenced efficient holding but, at the moment of release, the pain was again felt in the right lumbar region

- horizontal plane: testing of the extrarotation to the right once again reproduced pain in the right lumbar region; testing of the intrarotation sequence to the right showed a significant weakness as compared to intrarotation to the left.

The test of the sequences in sitting highlighted:

- frontal plane: isometric holding of the right lateromotion sequence reproduced right lumbar pain; isometric holding of the left lateromotion sequence was asymptomatic

- sagittal plane: isometric holding of the retromotion sequence was asymptomatic, whereas testing of the antemotion sequence was similar to that in standing as it evidenced effective holding but, at

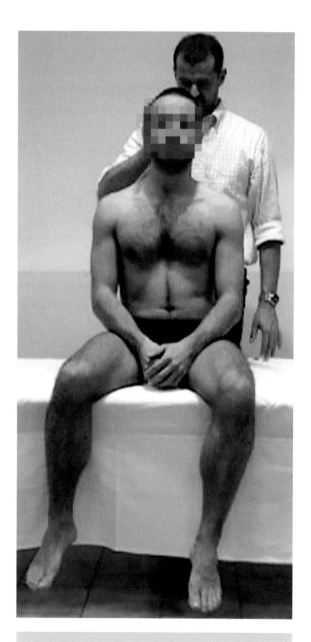

Figure 1.2
Test of the sequences in sitting. This test is similar to the test in standing. In this photograph it should be noted that, in the absence of contact with the ground, the subject tends to incline the lower limbs to the right, which is the side that is being activated in order to counteract the force applied by the physiotherapist

the moment of release, minor pain was also felt bilaterally in the lumbar region

- horizontal plane: testing of the extrarotation sequence was asymptomatic; similar to the test in standing, testing the sequence of intrarotation on the right highlighted significant weakness as compared to the left intrarotation sequence.

The results of MoVe are summarized in Table 1.1.

These results suggested that:

- all planes of movement presented painful and unstable elements; therefore, it was not possible to establish whether one plane was effectively worse than the others

- the involvement of the left lower limb was confirmed by the greater positivity of tests in standing as opposed to sitting; in particular, during the test for the right lateromotion sequence, pain referred along the right lower limb together with an incapacity of the left lower limb to counteract resistance

- the weakness found on intrarotation to the right, both in standing and sitting, indicated movement incoordination in the abdominal region, in relationship to the appendectomy scar

- the test of antemotion had an interesting outcome that is clinically rather frequent: the test was painful when the isometric load was released and the anterior part was relaxing. This type of response can be explained by an incoordination in the reciprocal inhibition of the two antagonist sequences, antemotion and retromotion. In other words, during activation of the antemotion myofascial sequence, the retromotion sequence was inhibited. However, when antemotion was relaxing, quick activation of retromotion to avoid the body falling forward caused the symptom to appear.

Palpation verification (PaVe)

The next step was palpation verification (PaVe). The centers of coordination (CC) and fusion (CF) in the lumbar segment (lu) were palpated first because this is where the main symptom was present.

The pelvis (pv) was the second segment chosen for palpation because of the surgical scar and because it was the segment that lumbar pain referred to. The left talus (ta), which was the other segment indicated from E.'s history, could have been an alternative choice for palpation.

The results of PaVe of the CC and CF are summarized in Table 1.2.

The aim of PaVe is always to choose a combination of altered points on a fascial structure (myofascial plane, diagonal, spiral) that require treatment.

The PaVe results called for further clinical reasoning:

- both unidirectional points (CC) and multidirectional points (CF) were involved; however, the altered CFs

Table 1.1						
	Frontal plane		Sagittal plane		Horizontal plane	
MoVe	LA rt	LA lt	RE	AN	ER	IR
Sequence tests – in standing	LU re–la rt*** (left leg instability)	—	LU re–la rt **	LU re–la rt** when relaxing	LU re–la rt **	LU an–la rt* (limited strength)
Sequence tests – in sitting	LU rt **	—	—	LU re bi * when relaxing	—	LU an–la rt* (limited strength)

Note: in FM asterisks from 1 (*) to 3 (***) rate the intensity of the pain and/or weakness reproduced during the test.

Table 1.2

Direction	AN		RE		LA		ME		ER		IR		AN-LA		RE-LA		AN-ME		RE-ME	
Segment	rt	lt	rt	lt	rt	lt	an	re	rt	lt	rt	lt	rt	lt	rt	lt	rt	lt	rt	lt
LU	*		**	*	**		*		*				*		**				*	
PV	**				***		**		**		*		**		*					

Note: in FM, 1 to 3 asterisks are used to indicate:
* pain on palpation
** pain on palpation associated with fascial tissue alteration
*** needle-like pain on palpation and/or referred pain associated with fascial tissue alteration.

Table 1.3

Points treated	la-lu rt	la-pv rt	an-la-pv 1 rt	me-ta-lt
Symptoms reproduced during treatment	Pain referred to posterolateral pelvic region	Densification dissolves rapidly	Intense pain that refers to posterolateral lumbar region	Needle-like pain, evident densification

(an-la-pv rt and re-la-lu rt) did not allow a clear identification of a diagonal or a spiral

- the right-sided position of both altered CFs did not suggest the involvement of a myofascial diagonal that could include the talus (ta) segment, given that the latter was located in the left lower limb
- as symptoms appeared both during unidirectional daily activities (e.g., getting up from an armchair) and worsened during sporting activities there was no clear indication for CCs as opposed to CFs
- tissue alterations were found on all planes, which confirmed the results of the MoVe.

Nevertheless, during PaVe the CCs appeared to be more altered on the frontal plane, which coincided with the MoVe results. The inability to sleep on the right side due to the lumbar pain was another coherent frontal plane sign. Therefore, the frontal plane was chosen for this first treatment.

1st treatment: frontal plane (Table 1.3)

MoVe immediately after treatment of the CC of la-lu on the right (la-lu rt) highlighted only a slight improvement in symptoms. Referred pain to the pelvis, reproduced during treatment of la-lu rt, indicated treatment of la-pv rt next, but post-treatment MoVe did not show any further significant improvement. Given the lack of change in symptoms and signs, I palpated other points on the frontal plane, including me-pv anterior and retro, la-ta and me-ta on the left. The me-pv points were not significantly altered and, while la-ta lt was altered and painful, me-ta lt was significantly worse in terms of densification and pain (***). The an-la-pv rt was also palpated again because, within the context of the FM biomechanical model, the ante-latero CF points in the trunk can be considered as coordinating elements for the frontal plane in the anterior quadrant (Figure 1.3). The right-sided CF of an-la-pv 1 was particularly densified, and palpation of this point referred pain to the posterior lumbar region. Treatment on this point proved to be extremely painful, with intense pain spreading both around the point and to the lumbar region, and several treatment pauses were necessary. Therefore, treatment of an-la-pv 1 rt was alternated with treatment of me-ta lt. Treatment of these two points required some modifications in the patient's position, which further allowed for pauses and relieved any positional tension due to antalgic contractions.

MoVe after treatment of these points highlighted a significant decrease in lumbar pain and a sensation of

Treatment of low back pain in a female athlete

Mirco Branchini

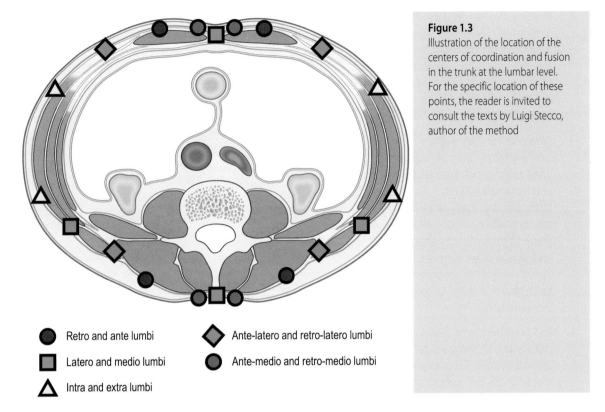

Figure 1.3
Illustration of the location of the centers of coordination and fusion in the trunk at the lumbar level. For the specific location of these points, the reader is invited to consult the texts by Luigi Stecco, author of the method

● Retro and ante lumbi

◆ Ante-latero and retro-latero lumbi

■ Latero and medio lumbi

● Ante-medio and retro-medio lumbi

▲ Intra and extra lumbi

lightness in the entire left lower limb. When palpated again, la-ta lt was no longer altered. This is a not infrequently encountered finding with this type of fascial work (see Discussion).

Results

The final post-treatment MoVe of the previously positive sequence tests showed significant improvement in all tests, with the absence of pain and increased stability when subjected to isometric holding. Only the test of the lateromotion sequence in standing highlighted some minor remaining instability. General movements, such as getting up from an armchair, were rated as 1/10 on the VAS.

E. was advised to avoid physically overloading her body in the following days and to return to sport gradually and she was warned that the treated areas could be sore up to 3 or 4 days after treatment.

A second session was programmed after 1 week but it was canceled because E. reported that her symptoms had further improved and that she had been able to return to her sporting activities without any pain.

Discussion

The results of this treatment highlight some important key aspects related to the biomechanical model of the fascial system, as proposed by Stecco, that physiotherapists should consider when applying FM:

1. The appearance of symptoms without a direct or traumatic cause is commonly related to previous events that can be revealed from the patient's history.

2. No matter how chronologically distant the events or topographically distant the body segments that emerge during history taking, each element of our body is always involved in a constant

interaction that regards the entire structure. This is not merely a holistic way of considering a person's disturbances, which for many other techniques may be considered almost a 'philosophy', but it is a truly mechanical requirement of the body as it attempts to compensate tension in order to guarantee optimal function.

3. Tensional compensations involving myofascial elements do not develop haphazardly. They respect the logic of biomechanical laws and dynamics (Stecco L. & Stecco A. 2017). In particular, for every action there is an equal and opposite reaction. When an element of a plane of movement is altered, there is almost certainly another element on the same plane, but working in the opposite direction, which will compensate in order to recreate a correct tensional balance.

4. Restoring tensional balance between antagonists is one of the principal objectives of every manual therapy. This case report demonstrates the logic of the antagonist activity between myofascial sequences. By referring to the FM biomechanical model, we can trace back to the dysfunctional myofascial elements, restoring their correct physiological state.

5. Movement and palpation verifications often present coherent indications. Treatment choices cannot be based entirely on palpation. All of the information collected during the initial anamnesis has to be considered. While the ascending or descending development of compensations can be misleading, the combination of movement and palpation verifications used in FM can help to clarify the direction of tensional compensations between past and presenting symptoms.

6. It is strongly recommended to temporarily discontinue treatment if a point is too painful, as occurred during the treatment of me-ta lt in this case report. Alternating deep friction with static pressure, interrupting treatment for some seconds and even moving to another point during these pauses are all tactics that can be employed to reduce treatment discomfort. At the same time, the tissue will begin to respond to the initial stimulus, which increases the local temperature. This response modifies the mechanical properties of the extracellular matrix (ECM) of the loose connective tissue found between fascial layers, presumably by setting off a reaction in the hyaluronan component of the ECM (Pavan et al. 2014). We can exploit this type of physiological response in order to reduce treatment time and patient discomfort.

7. In this case, a CC that was initially felt to be densified (la-ta lt) normalized after the treatment of an extremely altered antagonist CC (me-ta lt), which is situated in the medial crural fascia. While it is difficult to explain this reaction in neurophysiological terms, it is a phenomenon that occurs often during FM treatments, suggesting that FM could be a type of reflex therapy. Nevertheless, if we consider the reciprocal influence of the antagonist myofascial structures on tone within the same segment, it is plausible that alteration in one segment requires an equal and opposite response in the corresponding antagonist. Once treatment resolves tissue alterations, then this stimulus is removed and the antagonist element can be automatically normalized, without further intervention.

8. Even though the treatment reported in this chapter did not involve treatment of any internal dysfunctions, physiotherapists should keep in mind that the interaction between fascial tissues is not limited to musculoskeletal, tensional elements. By means of anatomical continuity, it also includes the tensional interrelationship between these elements and internal fasciae and organs. In particular, the fasciae of the trunk wall form a type of 'container' for the internal organs, and 'insertional fasciae' connect the internal organs to the musculoskeletal system (Stecco et al. 2017). Therefore, despite the apparent musculoskeletal characteristics of

presenting symptoms, our initial anamnesis should always include specific questioning with regards to internal dysfunctions (Stecco et al. 2017).

Conclusion

The interrelationship between distant segments, as described in this case report, is very frequent in daily clinical practice and it can also apply to other segments and conditions, such as scapulohumeral periarthritis that causes carpal tunnel syndromes, low back pain subsequent to whiplash, and so forth. On many occasions, investigations concentrate on the symptomatic segment and may even be supported by imaging (X-rays, computed tomography scans, MRI, or ultrasonography) of that same segment.

For this reason, it is very important that the hands of the physiotherapist make their own investigation, but with the added knowledge of what and where to investigate. As Luigi Stecco likes to say: 'a knowledgeable/skillful hand is powerful.'

References

Pavan PG, Stecco A, Stern R and Stecco C (2014) Painful connections: Densification versus fibrosis of fascia. Current Pain and Headache Reports 18 (8) 441. doi: 10.1007/s11916-014-0441-4.

Stecco L and Stecco A (2017) Manipolazione Fasciale® parte pratica – primo livello. Padua: Piccin.

Stecco C, Sfriso MM, Porzionato A, Rambaldo A, Albertin G, Macchi V and De Caro R (2017) Microscopic anatomy of the visceral fasciae. Journal of Anatomy 23 (1) 121–8.

EDITOR'S COMMENT

This chapter presents three different case reports involving treatments of centers of fusion arranged in myofascial spirals. The more superficial and middle myofascial layers include obliquely oriented collagen fibers that are tensioned by muscular insertions and are responsible for complex motion, such as spiral movements, and for the continuity between upper and lower limbs. This combination of obliquely arranged fascia and muscles forms anatomically identifiable myofascial spirals that can be traced from one foot to the contralateral shoulder. The cases include a baseball pitcher with right anterior shoulder pain and a history of metatarsal fractures in the left foot; a woman with a chronic limited left shoulder flexion sine causa and a history of recurrent sprains to the right ankle joint; and a woman with chronic pain and anteroinferior displacement of the right humeral head and a previous injury to her left ankle. The author, who is a Professor at the Tokyo Metropolitan University's Physical Therapy Department, introduced the Fascial Manipulation®–Stecco® method to Japan in 2011. He discusses how therapists need to examine the entire body, taking into consideration the myofascial sequences, diagonals and spirals in order to widen their range of treatment options.

Author's background

I completed my studies as a physical therapist in 1987 and then proceeded with a doctorate in anatomy in 2002. In 2008, I qualified as an Orthopedic Manual Physical Therapist (OMPT), a qualification that is recognized by the International Federation of Orthopedic Manual Physical Therapists (IFOMPT). Subsequently, I became a professor at the department of physical therapy working in the Graduate School of Human Sciences and Faculty of Health Sciences of the Tokyo Metropolitan University in 2012. It was at about this time that I became interested in the Fascial Manipulation®–Stecco® method (FM) and after completing all three levels of the FM training I qualified as a Level I and II teacher of this method in 2015. More recently, pursuing my passion for golf, in 2016, I qualified as a Golf Physical Therapist Official Instructor.

Experience with Fascial Manipulation®–Stecco® method

I came across the English publications of Luigi Stecco, in particular *Fascial Manipulation for Musculoskeletal Pain* (2004) and *Fascial Manipulation: Practical Part* (Stecco L. & Stecco C. 2009), and found them to be very interesting in their therapeutic proposals. I then accepted the challenge to translate these texts into Japanese. Following these publications in Japanese, we received a request from Italy regarding the possibility of Professor Carla Stecco performing a 1-day workshop in Japan to explain the theoretical basis of this method and to demonstrate the technique. I was directly involved in organizing this workshop, which was held in December 2011 and was well received by the numerous colleagues who attended.

Subsequently, I was able to travel to Italy to attend Level I in June 2012 at the international course held at the Stecco Medical Center. I returned to Italy in September 2012 for Level II and then completed Level III in September 2013. Level III proved to be more challenging, so I traveled yet again to Italy in September 2015 to repeat this course. Meanwhile, I translated many Stecco books from English to Japanese.

Since I have acquired my OMPT qualification, I have used many types of soft tissue mobilization, joint mobilization, and nerve mobilization techniques. However, as I began using FM, I found that the frequency of using these procedures dramatically decreased. This is because stretching and joint mobilization are often unnecessary due to the efficacy of FM.

There are times when I still use the Myofascial Release approach developed by John F. Barnes (1990), a physical therapist from the USA, particularly for people who are more sensitive to pain and athletes who have to play sport the day after treatment.

However, in fact, I often use FM, and my clinical methodology and reasoning have changed a lot since learning this approach. Even when I am holding an introductory workshop to FM there are inquiries from many therapists. In Japan, the fascial approach in general is having a significant expansion and there are waiting lists of colleagues who want to attend FM courses.

CASE REPORTS

Fascial Manipulation®-Stecco® method for dysfunctions extending from the foot to the contralateral shoulder

Three different cases involving treatments that incorporate centers of fusion (CFs) arranged in myofascial spirals will now be presented. Myofascial spirals involve the oblique fibers within the deep fascia and can be traced from one foot to the contralateral shoulder (Stecco L. & Stecco C. 2009).

Case 1

Introduction

A 21-year-old man, who had played hardball baseball as a pitcher in elementary, middle, and high school and currently plays softball baseball once a week at university, presented with pain in the right anterior shoulder region. He had been diagnosed as having a superior labrum anterior to posterior (SLAP) lesion of his right shoulder. He had undergone a calf exercise program for 6 months at another hospital, but his condition had not improved. Past medical history included stress fractures of the third and fourth metatarsal bones in his left foot 6 years earlier and he recalled that the pain had lasted for approximately 6 months. He had also developed a

right posterior elbow pain while pitching 4 years earlier, as well as a right anterior shoulder pain during the acceleration phase of pitching 1 year earlier.

Hypothesis

Extended pain from the stress fractures to the left third and fourth metatarsal bones, which had lasted for 6 months, was hypothesized as having prevented the patient from loading weight correctly on his left foot during the cocking and early acceleration phase of pitching. This could have prevented him from raising his right elbow above an imaginary line connecting the left and right shoulders (Figure 2.1), resulting in pain in the right elbow, progressing to involve the anterior aspect of his right shoulder.

Methodology

The apprehension test, which is a reliable orthopedic test used to assess the integrity of the shoulder joint or to check for instability (Kumar et al. 2015), highlighted pain in the right shoulder during flexion and

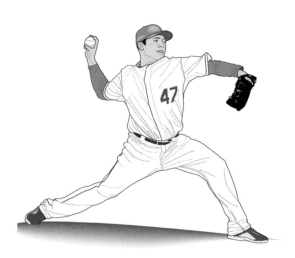

Figure 2.1
Incorrect pitching form with the elbow lower than the shoulder, or the line that joins the two acromions

lateral rotation. Reduced strength of shoulder medial rotators was also noted. Palpation verification (PaVe), performed according to FM procedure, revealed pain rated as 8 on a visual analog scale (VAS) in the regions of the CFs of retro-latero-pes (re-la-pe) on the left and retro-latero-cubitus (re-la-cu) on the right. In addition, VAS of 6 was reported on PaVe of ante-medio-scapula (an-me-sc) and ante-medio-humerus (an-me-hu) on the right, indicating an involvement of the retro-lateral myofascial spiral as described by L. Stecco and C. Stecco (2009) (Figure 2.2).

These findings suggested dysfunction extending in an ascending manner from the left toes, and also from the right elbow to the right shoulder.

Treatment: retro-lateral spiral (Table 2.1)

Post-treatment movement verification (MoVe) revealed pain relief and improvement in internal rotation strength of the right shoulder after treating the left re-la-pe CF point for approximately 4 minutes. Subsequently, treatment of the right re-la-cu, right an-me-sc, and right an-me-hu CFs increased the range of external rotation and further improved internal rotator strength of the shoulder.

Discussion

Interestingly, in this treatment, improvement in internal rotation strength of the right shoulder was seen immediately after treating the left re-la-pe CF point for approximately 4 minutes. In FM it is common to start treatment from a distant point that is related to a previous problem in order to verify one's initial hypothesis. Immediate post-treatment improvement in the presenting problem, in this case shoulder flexion, can reassure the therapist that the myofascial structure they have decided on is an appropriate choice. This rather distant connection can also be understood by analyzing the athletic gesture that this patient was required to perform. When playing baseball, it is necessary that a right-handed pitcher loads weight on their left leg in the cocking and early acceleration phases of pitching. When the elbow on the pitching side stays below the line

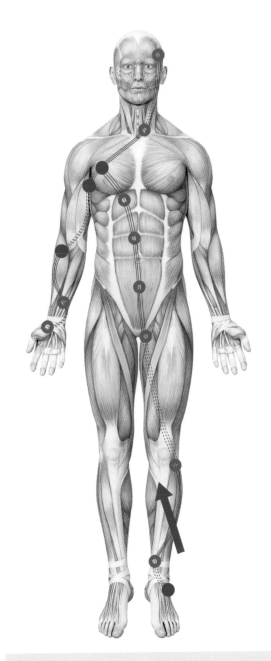

Figure 2.2
Retro-lateral myofascial spiral originating in retro-latero-pes (re-la-pe: red dot in the foot) and including retro-latero-cubitus (re-la-cu: red dot in the elbow region). The red dots represent the 4 points that were treated in Case 1

CHAPTER 2

Table 2.1				
Points treated: Case 1	re-la-pe lt	re-la-cu rt	an-me-sc rt	an-me-hu rt

connecting both acromions during these two phases, it is called a 'low elbow' and it is considered a faulty pitching pattern (Chalmers et al. 2017). This fault occurs frequently due to the onset of fatigue after throwing many balls. However, in the present case, the low elbow most probably occurred due to the inability to load weight correctly on the left leg, limiting the lateral rotation motion of the shoulder joint during the cocking phase and exerting excess valgus stress onto the elbow joint, which caused pain in the shoulder joint.

The patient had already undergone a general rotator cuff exercise program but no FM had been previously administered. Based on his previous history, and the low elbow during pitching, FM treatment directed at a myofascial spiral proved to be more effective. Despite a diagnosis of right SLAP lesion, it is important to assess and treat from the perspective of FM, which emphasizes the impact of previous injuries on the presenting symptoms.

Case 2

Introduction

A 22-year-old woman had been unable to perform more than 125° of left shoulder flexion for the last 2 years even though she had not had any direct trauma or strain to this shoulder. The passive end-feel of this movement was 'empty,' meaning that the pain prevented reaching end range of movement (ROM) due to protective muscle spasm. She complained of pain in the superior region of the left upper limb girdle, and also in the left chest and back areas, as well as the right thoracolumbar area, together with numbness in the left fourth and fifth fingers. Her past medical history (Table 2.2) included recurrent sprains to the right ankle joint, painful external tibial syndrome bilaterally, and bilateral anterior shin splints. Furthermore, the pelvis was elevated on the right side and tilted posteriorly and supination of the right foot was also noted.

Hypothesis

Pain in the left chest and back areas and right lumbar area suggested an involvement of CFs distributed along a myofascial spiral. This is because myofascial spirals pass from one side of the body to the other and tensional compensations that develop along these fascial structures follow this type of contralateral pattern. Moreover, recurrent sprains in the right ankle joint (see Table 2.2) were thought to be the cause of pain in the posterior side of the trunk and, conversely, shoulder flexion could be limited simply because it triggered pain in the posterior side of the trunk and therefore the patient had avoided this movement over the last 2 years.

Methodology

Movement verification (MoVe) highlighted shoulder flexion limited to 125°, which can be recorded as an-sc rt 125°. Palpation verification (PaVe) revealed pain rated 8 on the VAS in the right ante-medio-pes (an-me-pe) CF. This point was a silent CF, meaning that it was located in a currently asymptomatic area. Intense pain

Table 2.2 Relevant past medical history of case 2. Significant events have been placed on a timeline divided into years (Y) and starting from 11 years previous to first assessment				
11Y	10Y	3Y	2.5Y	2Y
Initial right ankle sprain	Severe right ankle sprain	Right ankle sprain	Bilateral anterior shin splints	Left shoulder joint flexion limitation: 125°

ranging from 6 to 8 on the VAS was also noted on palpation of retro-latero-talus (re-la-ta), retro-latero-coxa (re-la-cx), retro-latero-pelvis (re-la-pv), and retro-latero-lumbi (re-la-lu) on the right side and retro-latero-thorax (re-la-th), retro-latero-scapula (re-la-sc), and retro-latero-humerus (re-la-hu) on the left side, indicating a dysfunction involving the ante-medio spiral, as described by L. Stecco and C. Stecco (2009) (Figure 2.3). These findings suggested that the dysfunction of the right ankle joint also affected the left shoulder joint.

Numbness in the left fourth and fifth fingers was likely associated with the spiral connection between ante-medio-cubitus (an-me-cu), retro-latero carpus (re-la-ca), and ante-medio-digiti (an-me-di) on the left side.

Treatment: ante-medio spiral (Table 2.3)

Owing to the inclusion of the right an-me-pe, re-la-ta, and re-la-cx in the treatment, the ROM for left shoulder flexion increased to 150°. The treatment of the CFs of right re-la-pv, re-la-lu and left re-la-th, re-la-sc and re-la-hu further improved the ROM for left shoulder flexion to 180° and reduced pain from 8 to less than 3 on the VAS scale.

However, the patient explained that she no longer knew 'how' to flex her left shoulder because she had been unable to perform that movement for 2 years. Therefore, she underwent refresher exercises for the coordination of active movement and has maintained the improved range of motion to date.

Discussion

Recurrent sprains in the right ankle joint, painful external tibial syndrome bilaterally and bilateral anterior shin splints appeared to have caused compensatory ascending sensory disturbances in the centers of coordination (CCs) of the antemotion and mediomotion sequences. These sequences had possibly intertwined or combined to induce a dysfunction in the ante-medio myofascial spiral, which originates from the an-me-pe CF. As a consequence, pain and tension were induced in the thoracolumbar, chest, and dorsal regions of the body. Flexion of the left shoulder joint was limited because pain

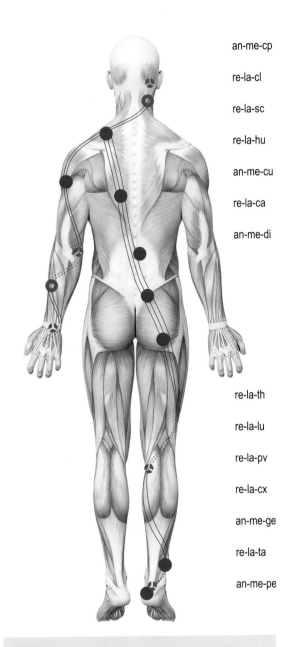

an-me-cp

re-la-cl

re-la-sc

re-la-hu

an-me-cu

re-la-ca

an-me-di

re-la-th

re-la-lu

re-la-pv

re-la-cx

an-me-ge

re-la-ta

an-me-pe

Figure 2.3
Ante-medio myofascial spiral originating in ante-medio-pes (an-me-pe: red dot in the foot). The other red dots represent points that were treated in Case 2

developed quickly in the right posterior side of the trunk whenever she attempted to perform this movement.

CHAPTER 2

Table 2.3				
Points treated: Case 2	an-me-pe rt	re-la-ta rt	re-la-cx rt	re-la-pv rt
	re-la-lu rt	re-la-th lt	re-la-sc lt	re-la-hu lt

It should be noted that shoulder flexion impairment can be caused by fascial densifications in the posterior region (retro) in addition to the anterior (ante) regions.

Case 3

Introduction

A 48-year-old woman began to feel sensations suggestive of anterior dislocation and depression of the right humeral head 2 years ago. In effect, the right humeral head was displaced in an anteroinferior direction. She complained of pain in the anterior and posterior aspects of the right shoulder with concomitant pain in the left pubic region. Her previous history included injury to the left ankle due to a car accident that had occurred 4 years earlier. As well as the left pubic region, she also had pain in the axillary region and the middle part of the upper arm on the right side.

Hypothesis

The patient had received treatment at various hospitals for about 2 years. These treatments only addressed the shoulder and the surrounding areas and while these treatments provided immediate relief, symptoms usually returned the following day. This suggested that the causal dysfunction was not in the shoulder joint, and a dysfunction within the myofascial structures was hypothesized. The condition suggested that an original dysfunction in the left foot could have spread to the contralateral right shoulder via tensional compensation within the myofascial spirals and/or sequences, possibly causing myofascial dysfunction in the CFs.

Methodology

Movement verification (MoVe) highlighted limited ROM for shoulder flexion, which was recorded as an-sc rt 140°. In addition, palpation verification (PaVe) revealed intense pain, ranging from 6 to 8 on the VAS scale, and tissue alteration in the CFs of retro-latero-pes (re-la-pe), ante-medio-talus (an-me-ta), ante-medio-coxa (an-me-cx) on the left and ante-medio thorax (an-me-th) and ante-medio- scapula (an-me-sc) on the right.

These findings suggested that through standing and walking, the dysfunction had progressed to involve the tissues around the left pubic bone and then to the right shoulder along the pathway of the retro-lateral myofascial spiral as a tensional compensation extending from the CF of re-la-pe on the left.

Treatment: retro-lateral spiral (Figure 2.4; Table 2.4)

Results

After treatment, pain in all CFs had reduced to a 3 on the VAS scale. At the second treatment session, the patient said: 'In the past, it didn't matter what kind of treatment I received; I was always left with a sensation that made me wonder if the shoulder was somehow dislocated. But this time, when I woke up the day after treatment, the sensation of dislocation in the right shoulder was gone. I was so surprised. It's as if I got my shoulder back. I am so happy.'

Discussion

In reference to the biomechanical model as presented by Stecco and increasing knowledge about fascial

Table 2.4			
Points treated: Case 3	re-la-pe lt	an-me-ta lt	re-la-ge lt
	an-me-cx lt	an-me-th rt	an-me-sc rt

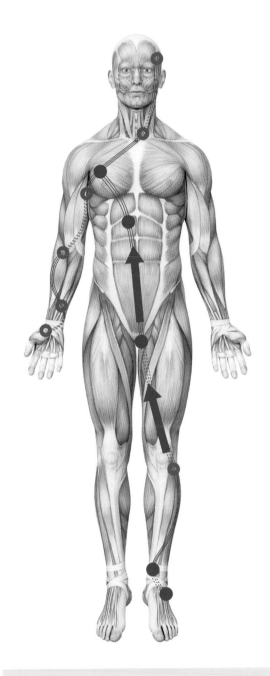

anatomy (Stecco C. 2015), it is possible to analyze what happened to this woman in the following way: due to the traumatic injury to the left ankle that the patient had sustained 4 years earlier, she was unable to load weight correctly on the left lower limb, which apparently led to the development of a gait with compensatory use of the adductor muscles of the left hip. Myofascial dysfunction of the adductor muscles disseminated to the lateral region of the left rectus abdominis, causing concomitant pain in the pubic region. This tension further spread to the attachment of the pectoralis major to the right side of the sternum, as well as the attachment of the right pectoralis major and minor to the ribs. Densification associated with points around the ankle region (left re-la-pe, left an-me-ta), and the pubic region where the adductors insert (left an-me-cx) generally remains unnoticed and is only detected as tenderness on palpation, making it easy for these points to become latent or silent CFs.

The patient received several forms of treatment at various hospitals; however, the focus was only on the shoulder and the surrounding areas. The following hypothesis was considered when attention was paid only to the shoulder: impaired dorsal gliding of the humeral head due to atrophy of the pectoralis major, pectoralis minor and latissimus dorsi, weakening of the subscapularis, impaired extension of the thoracic spinal facet joints, descent and impaired caudal slipping of the costovertebral joints, and dysfunction of the sternoclavicular and acromioclavicular joints. However, given that treatment to these areas did not yield lasting relief, this type of hypothesis proved to be invalid.

The range of treatment becomes much wider if the concept of CCs and CFs is incorporated into the hypothesis. Altered CCs within myofascial sequences and altered CFs along myofascial diagonals or spirals may be predicted or hypothesized based on the accompanying symptoms and the patient's past medical history, and an effective treatment approach may be established by verifying these hypotheses.

Figure 2.4
Retro lateral myofascial spiral originating in retro-latero-pes (re-la-pe: red dot in the foot). The other red dots represent points that were treated in Case 3

CHAPTER 2

Conclusion

It is important for therapists to examine the entire body, taking into consideration the myofascial sequences, diagonals and spirals. If pathological conditions persist after FM, then perhaps further investigations and specialized knowledge and skills are required. Otherwise, please keep in mind that, as therapists, we need to examine and treat not just local areas, but also the body as a whole.

References

Barnes JF (1990) Myofascial release: The search for excellence – a comprehensive evaluatory and treatment approach. Paoli: Rehabilitation Services, Inc.

Chalmers PN, Wimmer MA, Verma NN, Cole BJ, Romeo AA, Cvetanovich GL and Pearl ML (2017) The relationship between pitching mechanics and injury: A review of current concepts. Sports Health 9 (3) 216–21. doi: 10.1177/1941738116686545.

Kumar K, Makandura M, Leong NJ, Gartner L, Lee CH, Ng DZ, Tan CH and Kumar VP (2015) Is the apprehension test sufficient for the diagnosis of anterior shoulder instability in young patients without magnetic resonance imaging (MRI)? Annals of the Academy of Medicine, Singapore 44 (5) 178–84.

Stecco C (2015) Functional atlas of the human fascial system. Edinburgh: Churchill Livingstone, Elsevier.

Stecco L (2004) Fascial manipulation for musculoskeletal pain. Padua: Piccin.

Stecco L and Stecco C (2009) Fascial manipulation: practical part. Padua: Piccin.

Treatment of a street fighting, ex-professional boxer and Vietnam veteran – a complex case

3

Stephen F. Oswald, USA

EDITOR'S COMMENT

Patients with severe chronic pain can often respond relatively quickly to applications of Fascial Manipulation®–Stecco® method, suggesting that while it is a manual technique applied to peripheral soft tissue, it has a strong central nervous system component that is yet to be fully explained. This chapter, written in an accessible style that reflects the author's background, presents a complex case of chronic neck and arm pain with neurological signs that also involves prior cervical and ulnar nerve release surgery, as well as scarring from previous trauma and numerous abdominal surgeries. The author, a highly experienced doctor of chiropractic, uses narrative detail to document how the chronology of a person's musculoskeletal and biopsychosocial history can influence the therapist's choice of fascial structures to treat and the session-by-session clinical reasoning process that lies behind these choices.

Author's background

I started out in this profession nearly four decades ago, deep in the alleyways and mazes of Istanbul, under the guidance of a man who was a master with his hands and with herbs. But, to come back to the United States and practice what he was teaching me, I knew I needed a license. By a nice coincidence, a doctor of chiropractic from America befriended me, inspired me with his work, and off I went back to America. After nearly 6 years of postgraduate study, including my turning down an invitation with a full scholarship to attend a prestigious medical school, I became a doctor of chiropractic. For 32 years I have headed up two offices in America, one on Fifth Avenue in New York City and the other in the Upstate region. And for 25 of those years I had a small clinic in the poor section of Istanbul. My patient load includes elite level athletes, musicians, conductors, Wall Streeters, the whole gamut. The type of musculoskeletal injuries I treat includes everything one doesn't need to truly refer out to a surgeon. Prior to starting with Fascial Manipulation®–Stecco® method (FM), the soft tissue techniques that I applied included Graston, trigger point therapy, proprioceptive neuromuscular facilitation, transverse friction massage, and whatever else I picked up and made up along the way that worked. And a lot worked.

Experience with Fascial Manipulation®–Stecco® method

I first encountered FM through Dr Warren Hammer, a chiropractic physician of over 50 years' experience who refuses to stop learning and has done more good for the health of the human race via his teaching and clinical work than any other doctor I know. So, 6 years ago I found myself sitting in a New York airport hotel seminar room attending a class run by Dr Hammer and Dr Antonio Stecco. It was difficult stuff. But, after a couple of rounds of the same seminar and a lot of effort on transitioning to this technique, I think I've got it. Mostly, anyway. I think. Well, maybe not 40 percent yet.

The question that may come to mind is: why in heaven's name would a doctor with over 30 years of really doing a decent job of getting and keeping people healthy want to go through the hassle of learning a technique that is second to none in its degree of difficulty to learn? Maybe I should have spent my time mastering Swahili – I suspect it is a lot less difficult to master. Well, the short and succinct answer is, I was almost immediately in awe – in awe of a technique that I can only describe as inspired, but with a science base. If you think that is an oxymoron, you don't know FM.

Just what are the differences between this technique and the collection of stuff I made up and found along the way? And why did I choose this over Swahili? FM has a complexity and depth that allows it to be very nuanced. I now spend a good part of my working day in a state of deep

CHAPTER 3

'figuring-it-out' and almost all of the treatment time in what I term 'the zone' – a state of quiet, high concentration. It takes a lot of focus to stay in these small areas of altered tissue and to feel for the release, and to then decide where to go next. A patient described it by saying she felt the treatment as a mutual meditation. I like that, I think it is accurate. In the diagnosis phase, it has a near total disregard for the area of symptoms (except to rule out red flags and problems that are not treatable by soft tissue techniques). It has the same nearly total disregard for the area of symptoms when in the treatment phase – the symptomatic area is almost never treated – meaning it is cause-based, more so than any other technique I have ever used. This technique has a very good, though not absolute, science base to it. Take, for example, the study by Pintucci and co-workers (2017), showing some of the rationale behind the treatment of a rotator cuff tear with FM, or the study by A. Stecco et al. (2009) showing the continuity of the fascia and its attachments to the underlying muscles connecting the shoulder to the thumb, both mechanically and neurologically. It has dramatically changed the way I examine, diagnose, and treat a patient. So, I have significantly altered the routine I have evolved over the last 30 years. And I dislike change.

I have taken the seminars many times now. Why? To keep up with the current knowledge and fine tune my abilities? Yes. But really for the joy of being in the company of those I would consider a part of a historically very small group in the world that I label as 'Thinkers.' And I would add to that the modifier, 'Impassioned.'

Life has become more difficult for me since I chose to work with FM. Thanks. I now see patients that have more complex symptom pictures than any I had ever seen in the past three decades. I am sure there is a 'Most Complex Patient Ever Club' that meets weekly. They are highly organized. They send out scouts to various doctor's offices to get treated and then return to headquarters to report. If the treatment is successful, headquarters then sends out as many of their most complex of complex patients that they can, per week, to that office.

So here is a good example from 'The Club.'

CASE REPORT

Treatment of a street fighting, ex-professional boxer and Vietnam veteran

Introduction

C. arrived at my office accompanied by his son. He is a very well built, upright, well informed 70-year-old with a quick wit and a cache of interesting stories about his life in the Bronx. He is also a very involved grandfather. He was referred to me by an acupuncturist who is also certified in FM. C.'s past history includes two tours of active duty as a soldier in Vietnam (totaling 1 year of combat), semi-professional boxing and street fighting for many a decade in a tough neighborhood of New York City. In 1982, he was shot and severely injured and had undergone multiple abdominal surgeries as a consequence (Figure 3.1).

His presenting complaints were: left upper back pain and neck pain rated at an 8–9 on the visual analog scale (VAS) with 'numbness' type referral into first and second left fingers at a moderate to severe level, and with third finger numbness at a mild level. The pain began 15 plus years ago as a low-level pain but significantly increased at the end of the summer of 2016, despite the use of a hydromorphone and hydrocodone combination (derivatives of morphine and codeine, respectively). He had surgery in September of 2016, which included a laminectomy, removal of spurs, and discectomy of C3–4, C4–5, and C5–6. The pain continued unabated for several weeks post-surgery, decreased for a short period of time, then returned to its original, pre-surgical level. The pain further increased after a fall onto the left shoulder a few weeks before presentation. Complete pain relief occurs only for a few hours per day and only if he has had an acupuncture treatment that day and kept to his normal medication regime. Pain is provoked by most activities of daily living (ADL) and by left-side sleeping. Patient further states that no long-term significant improvement in pain occurs with medications – at times

Treatment of a street fighting, ex-professional boxer and Vietnam veteran – a complex case

Stephen F. Oswald

the pain can decrease to a 5–7 on the VAS scale. Visceral dysfunction is confined to constipation that is significantly relieved by the herb senna. Due to pain, the patient has done no significant exercise except walking.

Timeline

An important part of FM assessment is recording significant past trauma. Significant in this context refers to traumas that did not have a physiological healing or may have required extensive immobilization.

Significant past trauma for C. includes:

- Late 1960s: combat duty in Vietnam with relatively little physical damage. Nevertheless, extreme stress-based somaticized reactions could have led to an increase in baseline muscle tonicity (whose target areas are often the upper back and neck), creating the conditions for a later problem and, also perhaps, post traumatic stress disorder (PTSD)-related hyper-aggressiveness that led to increased street fighting and the possibly ultimate and predictable outcome – the shooting (Jakupcak et al. 2007)

- 1982: gunshot to abdominal area causing severe musculoskeletal damage as well as severe damage to colon, gallbladder, liver and lungs

- 1982–3: multiple abdominal surgeries to repair above stated organ systems (Figure 3.1)

- 1987: patella tendon surgery – left

- 1990: patella tendon surgery – right

- 2016: cervical discectomy, laminectomy, spur removal and the insertion of spacers: C3–4, C4–5, and C5–6 (Figure 3.2)

- 2016: left ulnar nerve displacement surgery to repair damage from incorrect placement of left arm during extended cervical surgery

- 2017: fall onto left shoulder with immediate and significant increase in pain level in presenting sites.

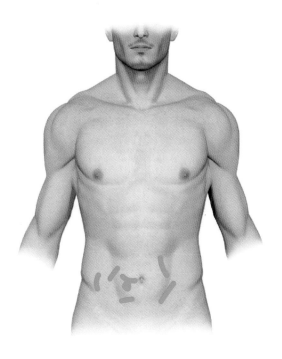

Figure 3.1
Illustration of the abdominal region highlighting scars (in green) caused by multiple abdominal surgeries to repair severe damage to the colon, gall bladder, liver and lungs following a gunshot wound in 1982

A consult with an orthopedist, including X-ray: no significant findings.

In this case report, assessment and treatment occurred in two different phases. In the first phase, the scapular segment was treated as part of the trunk. Why not as a limb? Simply because this pain began more than 15 years before the shoulder impact. So, it was hypothesized that the shoulder was merely an exacerbating factor. The presenting symptoms were not caused by the shoulder impact. Had I treated the scapular segment as a limb from the beginning, I certainly would not have found the involved segments.

CHAPTER 3

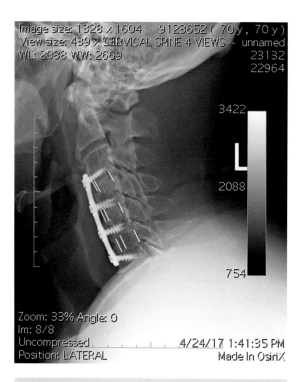

Image size: 1328 x 1604   9123652 (70y , 70 y)
View size: 439 x CERVICAL SPINE 4 VIEWS – unnamed
WL: 2088 WW: 2669   23132
                                           22964

3422

L

2088

754

Zoom: 33% Angle: 0
Im: 8/8
Uncompressed   4/24/17 1:41:35 PM
Position: LATERAL   Made In OsiriX

Figure 3.2
X-ray of the cervical spine taken after cervical discectomy, laminectomy, spur removal, and the insertion of spacers in the following intervertebral spaces: C3–4, C4–5 and C5–6 in 2016

Hypothesis: where is it all coming from, based on what I know so far?

If the left upper back pain and neck pain had decreased on lying down, I could safely assume the pain was coming from above – a 'descending' origin of pain – since the weight of the head would most likely be provoking the pain in the inferior areas. However, he does not have this decrease. We know that the older a significant injury is, the more time the patient's body has had to compensate. Further, regarding fascial damage, surgery is considered one of the most potentially damaging events for fascial layers. Surgery beats repetitive stress injury, chronic stress on the area and just about all trauma events – except possibly getting shot. So, combining the two – an old multiple surgery event with the gunshot event – allows me to hypothesize that the origin could be coming from below to up, therefore of 'ascending' origin: from the lumbar region to the neck and upper limb. Hence, for palpation verification (PaVe), my decision was to palpate the lumbar segment, being both a segment below the problem area (left upper back and neck) and one that sustained the most damage from the gunshot wound and subsequent related surgeries.

In order to identify a line (myofascial sequence, diagonal, or spiral), one must have two points. The second segment to palpate could be the symptomatic segment. In this case, scapula and collum were equally involved; therefore, I palpated both. I also performed PaVe on yet a fourth segment because a significant amount of densifications was found in the other segments.

Phase I

Movement verification

Movement verification (MoVe) of the neck (column: cl) and elbow (cubitus: cu) were chosen for assessment. Bilateral, lateral flexion of the neck (la-cl) showed that la-cl bilaterally provoked left-sided pain, with right la-cl provoking significantly more (left-sided) pain than left la-cl and allowing less lateral flexion than when moving to the left (essentially a positive left la-cl MoVe if looking at the movement outcome and a positive right MoVe if looking at the pain outcome).

Palpation verification

Palpation verification (PaVe), which is the most important part of the entire examination process, of the lumbar, collum and scapula segments highlighted the horizontal plane as the most involved plane, followed by the diagonal of retro-medio on the left.

Treatment of a street fighting, ex-professional boxer and Vietnam veteran – a complex case

Stephen F. Oswald

1st treatment: horizontal plane (Table 3.1)

I explained to the patient that the next day he might have an exacerbation of symptoms or tenderness over the points that were treated (see Discussion).

2nd treatment: horizontal plane (Table 3.2)

Status after first treatment: next day, a lot of pain. One really good day in the last 7 days since treatment, especially left upper back was helped a lot: 3 on VAS scale. Finger pain, no change. Still can't sleep. Night pain had decreased but it was 'not pain, just discomfort but just enough of it to keep me awake.'

Treatment of the horizontal plane continued, with the addition of centers of fusion in the thoracic region (Table 3.2).

Added: Graston of left transverse ligament, Sacro-Occipital Technique (SOT) for jammed sacroiliac joint.

3rd treatment: wherein an interesting experiment is performed (Table 3.3)

Status after second treatment: left finger numbness improved, regressed, improved again. Left cervical and upper back: a few good days, including 3 days without any severe pain; nights still bad.

I invited the referring acupuncturist to treat the centers of coordination that I had chosen for this session (Table 3.3).

Method and results of the experiment: the acupuncturist treated the points via multiple turnings and multiple insertions/removals of the acupuncture needles, finally leaving the needles in for 15 minutes. Ear points were included in the treatment regime. Upon removal of the needles, I found the densifications had completely dissolved in 3 of the 6 points and partially dissolved in the remaining three. I then completed the job, dissolving the remaining densifications and I added SOT II again, to continue the process of releasing the locked sacroiliac joint.

4th treatment (Table 3.4)

Status since last treatment: all generally good. Left hand and left lateral epicondyle: significantly decreased pain. Left upper back: VAS decreased from 8 to 5. Sleep pain still up and down but some nights are now pain-free.

Table 3.1 1st Treatment					
Points treated	er-sc lt	er-sc rt	ir-th lt	ir-th rt	ir-lu rt

Table 3.2 2nd Treatment					
Points treated	ir-sc lt & rt	ir-th lt & rt	er-cl lt & rt	er-lu lt	re-me-th 1, 2 lt

Table 3.3 3rd Treatment						
Points treated	er-th lt	er-lu lt	er-lu rt	ir-lu lt	ir-lu rt	ir-cl lt

Table 3.4 4th Treatment							
Points treated	er-sc lt	er-cp 3 lt & rt	er-cl lt & rt	er-th rt	re-la-th rt	re-la-lu rt (refers to wrist)	an-me-th lt

Note: treatment of er-sc lt was repeated as densification had not completely dissolved after the previous session.

5th treatment (Table 3.5)

Status after fourth treatment: decrease in 'nerve pain' (that is, left upper back, or the main presenting pain). Days without serious pain all day, for days at a time. No increase in medications. Anterior shoulder pain: acupuncture had stopped this until this morning, whereupon it returned. Left wrist good since first treatment until recently, whereupon pain returned but at a much lower level. Sleep improved, no interruption. Saw orthopedic surgeon, cervical specialist, who stated that no surgery is necessary and all the 'hardware' is in place.

Added: adjustment of left capita-lunate joint to improve the biomechanics in the wrist area.

Note: in this session I extended the treatment down into the left upper extremity.

6th treatment: spiral (Table 3.6)

Results after fifth treatment: daytime pain still much improved since treatment began (5–6 hours at a time without pain). However, there has been an exacerbation of nighttime left upper back pain, sometimes excruciating but sitting up for 5 minutes relieves pain. Daytime morphine now taken later in the day, sometimes skipping the second dose. Sleeping pain returns every half hour. Will see another orthopedist regarding the shoulder trauma.

Phase II

Results of phase I treatment

After a 10-week break from treatment, the patient states he feels generally better. He has gone from a VAS of 4–7 with medication and 8–9 between doses, to a more manageable level of pain in all of the symptom sites: cervical, upper back, shoulder, and wrist. He no longer takes his two doses of daytime morphine because of the decreased pain level, replacing them with just one Percocet (a combination of oxycodone and acetaminophen (paracetamol)). And since his nighttime pain is less, he has replaced his two doses of nighttime morphine with one Percocet pill, thus significantly reducing his total daily intake of opioids. He states he will soon be in contact with his medical doctor to begin the process of withdrawing from all of the pain medications.

Orthopedic and neurological tests and their improvement

Deep tendon reflexes (DTRs), which were originally within normal limits (WNL) bilaterally, had remained so. Dermatomes were originally WNL bilaterally excepting C6 and C7 on left, which were originally hypo and on re-evaluation had improved. Myotomes of shoulder shrug and shoulder abduction were WNL bilaterally and had remained so on re-evaluation. Elbow flexion was 3/5 SORT (strength on resistive testing), improving to 5/5 SORT, whereas elbow extension remains at 3/5 SORT. Both supination and pronation improved from 3/5 SORT to 5/5 SORT. Finger flexion and extension remains at 4/5 SORT.

In addition, patient reports continuing hypesthesia in left first and second finger.

Note: patient has had no acupuncture since third visit to this office but has had three physical therapy sessions consisting of passive stretches and simple exercises.

Hypothesis

I now wanted to consider the influence of the recent shoulder accident on the presenting symptoms. Why did I wait?

Table 3.5 5th Treatment							
Points treated	re-me sc rt	re-la-sc rt	re-la-cl rt	ir-hu lt	ir-sc lt	er-hu lt	er-sc lt

Table 3.6 6th Treatment			
Points treated	an-me-hu lt	re-la-sc lt	re-la-cu lt

Treatment of a street fighting, ex-professional boxer and Vietnam veteran – a complex case

Stephen F. Oswald

Consider the timeline: the presenting pain began 15+ years ago, increasing to a severe level in the summer of 2016, resulting in cervical surgery and a subsequent temporary decrease in pain, only to increase to a severe level soon after the surgery. I had two dramatic traumas to consider: first the gunshot wound and then the cervical surgery (followed by a second surgery for the ulnar nerve damage). Of these traumas, the most important to consider was the gunshot since this is the only trauma that occurred before the presenting pain began. Further, since pain on presentation did not decrease in non-weight-bearing positions such as supine, prone, or side-lying, I hypothesized that this pain did not have a descending cause, that is, coming from the neck and going downward. However, I duly noted that the impact on the left shoulder caused an immediate and significant increase in pain level so, eventually, it had to be addressed. The shoulder injury was a major, very recent, exacerbating influence, not the cause. The presenting pain began many years before the shoulder injury. In summary, since it is a major influence, when the causal segments are sufficiently treated, this influence should be addressed.

7th treatment: frontal plane (Table 3.7)

Chiropractic adjustment to left capita-lunate joint and to left glenohumeral joint were also performed.

Discussion

After the first treatment, I always explain to the patient that during the following days they may have an exacerbation of symptoms or tenderness over the treated points. This is presumably due to the influx of a combination of proinflammatory molecules and hyaluronidase triggered by treatment (Stern & Jedrzejas 2006).

Being a chiropractic physician, I also utilized chiropractic adjusting techniques to restore the biodynamics of the joints. In C.'s case, because of the fragility and pathology of the joints, I only adjusted the wrist and pelvis.

I frequently re-tested the previously identified faulty MoVes and consistently found them improved, if only slightly. In my work, I also use multiple orthopedic tests including deep tendon reflexes, dermatomes, myotomes and muscle testing. FM has changed my interpretation of many of these tests. Take the example of the sciatic neural stressing tests (Straight Leg Raise, Sicard's, Bragard's, etc.): classically, a positive test supports a sciatic neuritis, possibly herniated disc based. However, a newer, fascial based hypothesis opens up the possibility that a fascial pathway along the posterior lower limb is in a state of compensatory 'over-glide' because of a state of 'under-glide' somewhere along the posterior of the limb. This will potentially convert the mechanoreceptors present in the fascia into nociceptors, thus causing a pain along and in that posterior fascial pathway. I may well treat the disc, but I will also treat the fascia to remove the over-glide, thus allowing the nociceptors to convert back to proprioceptors. (Note: even if the basis for the sciatic pain – or sciatic-like pain – is a herniated disc, because of the intimate relationship between the discs and the fascia, FM may well also aid in reducing the herniation.)

I must note here the patient has become a much more engaged person, wanting to share several stories of combat in Vietnam. It is possible that our work together has lifted enough of the pain that encompassed his everyday thought process, filtered every thought and action; that the tremendous emotional trauma that occurred to him on the battlefield got lost in the muddle of pain and painkillers. As the physical pain lifts, as the fog of heavy painkilling drugs lifts, as he trusts me more, he is able to see the battlefield once again and talk about it. Just a thought – more of a hope really. Probably not true. It would make for a great story though.

The patient self-discharged after the last treatment. Perhaps he felt he had gone far enough in his treatment. He was a very self-sufficient person. My experience is that some patients ask for help only to get the healing started, and then they leave the program when they feel this has occurred, to let their bodies work out the problem, returning for a regular fine-tuning or, if the healing plateaus, for a kickstart. Stay tuned.

Table 3.7 7th Treatment		
Points treated	la-sc lt	me-hu lt

CHAPTER 3

References

Jakupcak M, Conybeare D, Phelps L, Hunt S, Holmes HA, Felker B, Klevens M and McFall ME (2007) Anger, hostility and aggression among Iraq and Afghanistan war veterans reporting PTSD and sub-threshold PTSD. Journal of Traumatic Stress 20 (6) 945–54.

Pintucci M, Simis M, Imamura M, Pratelli E, Stecco A, Ozcakar L and Battistella LR (2017)

Successful treatment of rotator cuff tear using Fascial Manipulation® in a stroke patient. Journal of Bodywork and Movement Therapies 21 (3) 653–7.

Stecco A, Macchi V, Stecco C, Porzionato A, Ann Day J, Delmas V and De Caro R (2009)

Anatomical study of myofascial continuity in the anterior region of the upper limb. Journal of Bodywork and Movement Therapies 13 (1) 53–62.

Stern R and Jedrzejas MJ (2006) Hyaluronidases: their genomics, structures and mechanisms of action. Chemical Reviews 106 (3) 818–39.

Treatment for temporomandibular dysfunction in a patient with juvenile arthritis

Angela Mackenzie, Canada

4

EDITOR'S COMMENT

Registered massage therapists who combine massage therapy with movement-based approaches to patient rehabilitation are finding that they can successfully integrate the Fascial Manipulation®–Stecco® method into their work. The author of this chapter is a registered massage therapist and owner of a successful massage therapy clinic who has been studying this method since 2011. She presents a case report regarding the treatment of myofascial jaw pain, headache, and migraines in a 36-year-old man who was diagnosed with juvenile arthritis when he was 3 years old. After treating the patient once a month for 4 months, an overall reduction in pain and a reduction in pain medication was evident. These results were reported to be maintained at a 1 year follow-up. The author observes another positive outcome of this method is the reduced necessity of working directly in the area where the patient perceives pain.

Author's background

I completed my Registered Massage Therapist diploma in 1995 from the West Coast College of Massage Therapy in Vancouver, in British Columbia, Canada. My previous work as a dental assistant fostered my special interest in jaw pain and dysfunction. My work experience from 1999 to March 2004 was in a large physiotherapy clinic where I learned to combine massage therapy with movement-based approaches to patient rehabilitation. In September 2004 I moved to Toronto, Ontario, and broadened my work experience at a sports medicine clinic and as a teaching assistant at the Canadian College of Massage and Hydrotherapy. In 2005 I returned to Vancouver, where I opened a successful massage therapy clinic. I also completed intraoral and extraoral studies and certification in Washington State, USA.

Experience with Fascial Manipulation®–Stecco® method

I first became interested in Fascial Manipulation®–Stecco® method (FM) in 2010 and began a course of study in the method in Vancouver in 2011. The methodology, and the books and research studies produced by the Stecco family, have provided a deeper understanding of 'fascia' and its potential role in body movement and overall health. I completed Level I, II and III FM courses by June 2015 and use the method in my practice daily. FM has informed how I approach patient history questions, movement assessment, and my palpation skills. The manual application considers the whole body and attention is focused on improving movement with reduced pain.

Future learning interests will include studies in the area of fascia and its relationship to the nervous system and reconciling the role of fascia and its contribution to pain.

Introduction

Temporomandibular dysfunction (TMD) and the diagnosis of myofascial pain are common in adults with juvenile arthritis. These symptoms are often accompanied by tension-type headaches or migraines. Also, it is important to note that not all presentations have joint or movement anomalies, yet symptoms persist and can be difficult to diagnose or classify.

The term temporomandibular dysfunction (TMD) is used to describe a population of patients with myofascial symptoms causing abnormal, usually painful, function of the masticatory muscles, joints, and condyle–disc complex. These symptoms are not always directly related to temporomandibular joint (TMJ) function (Larheim 2005). Individual patients with TMD can have distinct variations of symptoms and different mechanisms for their disease. Symptoms can include chronic headaches, migraines, tooth pain, bruxism, and head and neck muscle tension, all due to the close anatomical and physiological relationships (Giamberardino et al. 2007).

For the purposes of this study it was also observed that common mechanisms of TMD are the inflammatory arthritides, and in particular, juvenile arthritis (Engström et al. 2007; Carrasco 2015).

The complexity of myofascial symptoms makes TMD difficult to define or classify (Brandlmaier et al. 2003) because all these symptoms are common patient complaints associated with soft-tissue injuries or causative factors.

Treatment of TMD can vary, from medicine to dental appliances, bite alterations, trigger point and botulinum toxin injections, as well as dry needling, massage, physiotherapy, and low amplitude thrust techniques (Butts et al. 2017). While most methods show efficacy in reducing symptoms, some can be invasive, expensive, or not easily accessible for the patient.

CASE REPORT

Massage therapy treatment for temporomandibular dysfunction in a patient with juvenile arthritis

The aim of this study is to assess whether FM, a manual massage method, is an effective conservative treatment approach for the treatment of myofascial jaw pain in a patient with juvenile arthritis.

This case concerns a Caucasian male diagnosed with juvenile arthritis at the age of 3 years. Now 36 years old, he presents with TMD symptoms of jaw pain, headache, and migraines. An initial medical treatment approach that included trigger point injections was effective but was also perceived by the patient to be painful and invasive.

Methodology

i. Patient history

The patient in this study, J., is a 36-year-old male who was diagnosed with juvenile arthritis (JA) at 3 years of age in 1984. He presented with pain and stiffness in multiple joint areas: bilateral masticatory muscles (right more than left), bilateral neck, right elbow bursitis, and right knee. Chronic weekly headaches ranged in frequency and severity and were rated on the visual analog scale (VAS) as between 3 and 6. They could start to cluster and progress to migraines of VAS 7–9, which J. experienced at least once a month. The patient reported that headache, jaw pain, and muscle tension seemed to be related but were not exacerbated by movement, eating or talking. Jaw symptoms arose sporadically and were not necessarily present in the morning or evening.

To manage these symptoms, he was prescribed a number of medications (Table 4.1, left column) and was receiving monthly trigger point injections, first of saline and then of lidocaine, from an oral pain specialist. The trigger point injections were in the temporalis and masseter musculature bilaterally. This treatment was reducing the frequency and severity of headaches, migraines, and also controlling temporomandibular dysfunction (TMD) symptoms. Nevertheless, J. researched and requested massage therapy as an alternative treatment to trigger point injections. Massage therapy is perceived by the patient to be less painful and more easily accessible.

ii. Observation

The patient uses a cane in his left hand, and has an antalgic gait leaning to the left side in the first part of the gait phase and then shifting to the right side. He has limited dorsiflexion in the right ankle. He wears glasses and has poor eyesight.

iii. Movement verification

TMJ range of motion was measured in millimeters (maximum mouth opening, protrusion, right and left laterotrusion) and all movements were within normal range.

Treatment for temporomandibular dysfunction in a patient with juvenile arthritis

Angela Mackenzie

iv. Palpation verification

A bilateral palpation of muscles of mastication was performed as indicated by FM guidelines.

v. Neurological or referred pain

Cervicogenic pain and headaches are recurrent, 1–2 per week and occasionally of a cluster-type, which worsen in severity and progress to migraines 1–2 per month. Migraines are sporadic and can happen any time of day.

vi. Special tests

TMJ range of motion is within the normal range for all planes of movement; therefore, no X-rays or MRI (magnetic resonance imaging) was ordered by the oral pain specialist. I used a 10-point VAS scale for pain levels, with 0 being the absence of pain and 10 being the worst pain ever.

The initial presentation was jaw and head pain VAS 6, with headaches ranging from VAS 3 to 6. For migraines the VAS was 6–8 out of 10. VAS pain levels were assessed in the pre- and post-treatment phase of each FM session (Figure 4.1).

vii. Treatment

FM treatment sessions were 45 minutes in duration, on a monthly basis for 4 months. I have 6 years of experience using this method and I performed all FM sessions. Areas of treatment are illustrated in Figures 4.2 and 4.3. The choice and number of specific sites for manipulation were determined on the basis of the FM assessment guidelines and also the needs of the patient. In FM, the manual technique is applied by use of digital pressure exerted by the therapist over specific centers of coordination (CC) points or center of fusion (CF) points. I used my knuckles or fingertips to exert the pressure on the fascia of the illustrated muscular areas.

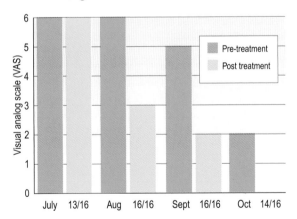

Figure 4.1
Monthly treatment dates are indicated along the bottom with pre- and post-treatment VAS pain scores. On October 14, 2016, the patient had no headache or jaw pain post treatment and, at October 2017 follow-up, symptom management had been maintained for 1 year

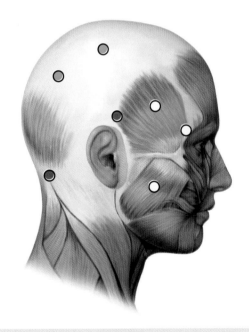

Figure 4.2
Right view: center of coordination (CC) and fusion (CF) points treated with Fascial Manipulation® technique by Luigi Stecco. White circles = points on the frontal plane; red circles = points on the horizontal plane; green circles = retro-medio (CF) points

CHAPTER 4

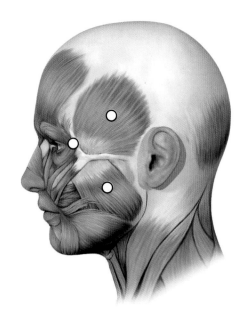

Figure 4.3
Left view: centers of coordination used in treatment for temporomandibular dysfunction. White circles = points on the frontal plane

viii. Medications

In the table of medications (Table 4.1), the column on the left is a list of prescribed medications that the patient was taking at the beginning of treatment. The column on the right lists the medications needed at discharge on October 14, 2016, after four treatment sessions of FM.

A follow-up with the patient confirms medications in the second list have remained consistent for a year.

Results

Maximum pain levels on a VAS demonstrate that massage therapy by way of the FM method appears to be equally effective in the outcome parameters at a 4-month and then a 1-year follow-up (see Figure 4.1). Furthermore, a significant reduction in the use of pain medication was seen at a 1-year follow-up (see Table 4.1). These findings are consistent with literature that supports the effectiveness of conservative treatment approaches to myofascial pain of the head, neck, and jaw muscles.

Discussion

The therapeutic effects of intraoral and extraoral manual therapy and self-care management of TMD have been demonstrated in a number of randomized control trials and systematic reviews (von Piekartz & Hall 2013; Randhawa et al. 2015; Martins et al. 2016). FM is a manual therapy method developed by physiotherapist Luigi Stecco to treat myofascial pain in the body and it has been shown to be effective for TMD (Guarda-Nardini et al. 2012).

Studies of fascial anatomy, histology, and physiology are changing our understanding of the role of fascia and myofascial pain. With FM, L. Stecco (2004) hypothesizes that the myofascial system is a three-dimensional continuum with a comprehensive, functional role in musculoskeletal activity and dysfunctions. Musculoskeletal

Table 4.1 Prescribed medications needed before and after October 14, 2016	
Medications before October 14, 2016	Medications after October 14, 2016, and at 1-year follow-up*
Nabilone 1 mg	N/A
Gabapentin 100 mg	N/A
Celebrex® (celecoxib) 200 mg	Celebrex® (celecoxib) 200 mg
Actemra® (tocilizumab) 2 shots per month	Actemra® (tocilizumab) 2 shots per month
Diclofenac as needed	N/A

N/A = not applicable or no longer taken.
*At one-year follow-up the patient confirmed that medications in the second list had remained consistent for one year.

Treatment for temporomandibular dysfunction in a patient with juvenile arthritis

Angela Mackenzie

dysfunction is considered to occur when the muscular fascia no longer slides, stretches, and adapts correctly. Given that deep fascia is generally formed by two to three layers of parallel collagen fiber bundles with different orientations, and that each layer is separated from the adjacent one by loose connective tissue (Stecco C. et al. 2008), the rationale for using the technique is based on the capability of fascial tissues to slide in relation to surrounding tissues. The mechanical load exerted by the therapist over a specific center of coordination (CC) or center of fusion (CF) point provokes a localized hyperemia that may affect the ground substance of the loose connective tissue component found in retinacula or the deep fascia, restoring gliding between fiber layers and allowing a new tensional adaptation throughout the fascial system.

A benefit of using the method is that the therapist often does not work in the area where the patient perceives pain, known in this method as the center of perception (CP), but above or below these sites.

Some interesting studies question whether fascia can affect pain (van der Wal 2009) or biomechanics (Proske & Gandevia 2009). The associated manual therapy method and whether it can have a therapeutic effect warrants further study, but there is some evidence recognizing that conservative physical therapies, including massage, reduce head and neck pain (Racicki et al. 2013).

Conclusion

Future long-term group studies recognizing the benefits of massage therapy and other conservative approaches to TMD in the presence of juvenile arthritis would be beneficial.

FM is a good treatment of choice for the soft tissue structures involved in TMD and that translates clinically into improved proprioception, motor control, and decreased experience of pain. Another area of interest is the contextual effect massage therapy has on patients with jaw pain. This case demonstrates a patient's perception of massage to be less invasive and less painful than injections. The biopsychosocial aspects of TMD are notable and include physiology, emotions, behaviors, and beliefs.

References

Brandlmaier I, Grüner S, Rudisch A, Bertram S and Emshoff R (2003) Validation of the clinical diagnostic criteria for temporomandibular disorders for the diagnostic subgroup of degenerative joint disease. Journal of Oral Rehabilitation 30 (4) 401–6.

Butts R, Dunning J, Pavkovich R, Mettille J and Mourad F (2017) Conservative management of temporomandibular dysfunction: A literature review with implications for clinical practice guidelines. Journal of Bodywork and Movement Therapies 21 (3) 541–8.

Carrasco R (2015) Juvenile idiopathic arthritis overview and involvement of the temporomandibular joint: Prevalence, systemic therapy. Oral and Maxillofacial Surgery Clinics of North America 27 (1) 1–10.

Engström AL, Wänman A, Johansson A, Keshishian P and Forsberg M (2007) Juvenile arthritis and development of symptoms of temporomandibular disorders: A 15-year prospective cohort study. Journal of Orofacial Pain 21 (2) 120–6.

Giamberardino MA, Tafuri E, Savini A, Fabrizio A, Affaitati G, Lerza R, Di Ianni L, Lapenna D and Mezzetti A (2007) Contribution of myofascial trigger points to migraine symptoms. Journal of Pain 8 (11) 869–78.

Guarda-Nardini L, Stecco A, Stecco C, Masiero S and Manfredini D (2012) Myofascial pain of the jaw muscles: Comparison of short-term effectiveness of botulinum toxin injections and fascial manipulation technique. Cranio 30 (2) 95–102.

Larheim TA (2005) Role of magnetic resonance imaging in the clinical diagnosis of the temporomandibular joint. Cells Tissues Organs 180 (1) 6–21.

Martins WR, Blasczyk JC, Aparecida Furlan de Oliveira M, Lagôa Gonçalves KF, Bonini-Rocha AC, Dugailly PM and de Oliveira RJ (2016) Efficacy of musculoskeletal manual approach in the treatment of temporomandibular joint disorder: A systematic review with meta-analysis. Manual Therapy 21 10-7.

Proske U and Gandevia SC (2009) The kinaesthetic senses. Journal of Physiology 587 (17) 4139–46. doi: 10.1113/jphysiol.2009.175372.

Racicki S, Gerwin S, DiClaudio S, Reinmann S and Donaldson M (2013) Conservative physical therapy management for the treatment of cervicogenic headache: A systematic review. Journal of Manual and Manipulative Therapies 21 (2) 113–24. doi: 10.1179/2042618612Y.0000000025.

Randhawa K, Bohay R, Côté P, van der Velde G, Sutton D, Wong JJ, Yu H, Southerst D, Varatharajan S, Mior S, Stupar M, Shearer HM, Jacobs C and Taylor-Vaisey A (2015) The effectiveness of noninvasive interventions for temporomandibular disorders: A systematic review by the Ontario Protocol for Traffic Injury Management (OPTIMa) collaboration. Clinical Journal of Pain 32 (3) 260–78. doi: 10.1097/AJP.0000000000000247.

Stecco C, Porzionato A, Lancerotto L, Stecco A, Macchi V, Day JA and De Caro R (2008) Histological study of the deep fascia of the limbs. Journal of Bodywork and Movement Therapies 12 (3) 225–30.

Stecco L (2004) Fascial manipulation for musculoskeletal pain. Padua: Piccin.

van der Wal J (2009) The architecture of the connective tissue in the musculoskeletal system – an overlooked functional parameter as to proprioception in the locomotor apparatus. International Journal of Therapeutic Massage and Bodywork 2 (4) 9–23.

von Piekartz H and Hall T (2013) Orofacial manual therapy improves cervical movement impairment associated with headache and features of temporomandibular dysfunction: A randomized controlled trial. Manual Therapy 18 (4) 345–50. doi: 10.1016/j.math.2012.12.005.

Is this method magic? Certainly not. Three case reports

Eran Mangel, Israel

EDITOR'S COMMENT

The author of this chapter sees himself as coming from the practitioner's standpoint rather than from a purely academic background. After more than 30 years of full-time clinical practice as a physiotherapist, including treating top-level athletes in first division teams, he uses his practitioner's perspective to discuss three cases of people who came to his clinic with little hope and a lot of suffering and went home with better function and a smile. These three cases have all been treated with the musculoskeletal approach and include a young woman with severe ankle instability sine causa who had falling and balance problems, an elderly man with debilitating back pain that had limited him to moving with a wheelchair, and a young athlete who could no longer run because of a 'runner's knee.' As applied in these three cases, the successful combination of Fascial Manipulation®–Stecco® method treatments with suitable exercise regimens is a recurrent theme throughout this book. Working on key fascial points to correct sliding of fascial tissues can seemingly reduce pain on movement, restore appropriate proprioceptive information, and permit efficient muscle fiber recruitment, thereby enhancing targeted exercise programs.

Author's background

I graduated from Tel Aviv University in 1986 as a physiotherapist (BPT) and worked in the public sector for 9 years before beginning my career in private practice. My first clinic was very small, but my career developed and since 2006 I have been one of the three owners of Medix, which is the biggest private sports medicine center in Israel, where I am also head of the physiotherapy department.

For the last 22 years, I have worked with different sports clubs and first division football, basketball (men and women), and handball teams, and in diverse clinics, treating all kinds of orthopedic injuries and conditions. I was born in 1958, I am married with four children, and I consider myself a family man. I am a lifetime athlete, a marathoner, and several times Ironman 'finisher' and I enjoy the toughness of the challenge.

During the 31 years of my career, I have gathered knowledge from quite a few postgraduate courses, including Maitland's spinal and peripheral mobilization, the Cyriax concept, the Mulligan concept and many more enriching courses and professional conventions.

I tend to doubt my clinical results and I understand that we can never know enough about our profession. Nevertheless, I wake up every morning blissful to meet new challenges.

Experience with Fascial Manipulation®–Stecco® method

My Fascial Manipulation®–Stecco® method (FM) studies started in 2011 and I have completed Level I, II, and III training. Before encountering the FM method, my treatment basically focused around and on the affected area alone. I did not take into consideration the influence of remote bodily disabilities and lack of mobility, nor did I look at the body as a whole, so that has been a major change in my approach.

Another element that was missing prior to using FM was the connection between cause and effect and trying to identify this relationship even prior to commencing any treatment. I now begin this type of analysis during the interview that precedes the physical examination.

Introduction

Theoretical framework

The anatomical significance of the fascial layers and knowledge concerning them has advanced in the course

CHAPTER 5

of recent years (Findley 2011). After long years of referring to this tissue as being of lesser importance and as a merely passive one, in the last 30 years or so this opinion has changed completely.

The fascial layers and their dynamic value have become important and have turned into an effective treatment target (Stecco L. 2004). The 'hands-on' physiotherapist and more manual therapists who have been exposed to the FM® method have gained an effective tool and a new way of approaching pain and dysfunction (Pavan et al. 2014).

A few questions do still emerge, for example: is the physical information we are getting from this tissue important? Are the orthopedic and neurologic data that have been connected with this tissue meaningful or just esoteric? Clinical research regarding FM is increasing (Picelli et al. 2011; Branchini et al. 2016; Kalichman et al. 2016) and in years to come it will grow and undoubtedly will be able to provide us with more and more answers and evidence. Meanwhile, we should use all the information we can gather from the body, and from our patients in general, in order to treat the somatic and visceral dysfunctions that we are presented with.

What is missing?

I am not a person from a purely academic background. I am coming from the practitioner's perspective and, even though I read a lot and am learning all the time, I necessarily take the practitioner's side. In my personal philosophy, the best way to treat encompasses two main fields: learning and trying. When we try we make mistakes and then we learn from them, and this is the way to become a better physiotherapist. Nevertheless, on our way to treating successfully, referring to academic publications and using our understanding based on smart and mindful experience is essential, and this approach will lead us to the best possible outcome.

During more than 30 years of being a full-time physiotherapist, my capacity to assess efficient treatment techniques has mostly come from my patients and the way they have reacted to my treatments. This is why you will not see charts or statistics related to the case reports I am presenting, nor scientific biology and movement analysis. On the other hand, I will discuss people who came to the clinic with little hope and a lot of suffering, and went back home with better function and a smile.

Work method

When a patient is coming for treatment, in order develop the best clinical reasoning and to make the best functional diagnosis, we need to gather all the medical information about them that we can.

When applying the FM method, first and foremost comes the interview, which consists of listening to the patient and is such an important part of the meeting. As Sir William Osler, a renowned Canadian physician, once said: 'Listen to the patient, he is giving you the diagnosis'. Therefore, all information is important and should be considered.

Understanding the patient's history is of the utmost significance, and the phrase 'Old is gold' is as important as the severity of past injuries, traumas, and surgeries. Basically, we need to take into account all possible factors that can influence the present injury and dysfunction. In the past, it was sometimes confusing when a patient presented with multiple complaints in different body areas. Now we can use the Stecco model to achieve a better understanding of the problem.

The term 'dysfunction' is used in order to distinguish it from the term 'pathology.' The physiotherapist can repair the first but should let the medical doctor take care of the latter. As soon as we have recognized the pattern of the past injuries or pain and the association with the present dysfunction, the physical examination and assessment start in order to determine the best treatment. As we know, the body can be divided into three dimensions and, for the purpose of treatment, each one has a sub-dimension.

Given that the structure of the fascial layers is distinct and relatively accurate (Stecco C. 2015), it is possible to

Is this method magic? Certainly not. Three case reports

Eran Mangel

identify a sequence of FM points located within a fascial structure (plane, diagonal, spiral, tensile structure, catenary, or even a superficial fascia quadrant) to get the best results from any given single treatment. Obviously, the results can also depend on additional factors, such as inappropriate habits and incorrect body movements, and not only on the treatment, and these factors should also be taken into consideration when developing a treatment plan.

CASE REPORTS

In this chapter, I will describe three cases in which I have used the viewpoint, understanding, and techniques that I have learned from studying the FM method, as presented by Luigi Stecco, his family and collaborators, and their research.

The causes of the injuries differ from one case to another but the FM approach made them all easy to deal with.

These three cases include a young lady who had ankle instability for no obvious reason and had falling and balance problems; an elderly man with back pain that caused him to need to be pushed in a wheelchair by his children; and a young athlete who could not run because of a 'runner's knee.'

I will show you how I approached these different problems, in these diverse age groups, by following the guidelines of the FM method, and how the solutions were surprising. It is very encouraging to note that these types of pain and dysfunction can be reversed and that we can restore ability, function, and self-confidence.

Case 1: chronic ankle instability leading to recurrent falls

M. is a 22-year-old student. She came to my clinic with her mother and the first thing she said to me before I even asked a question was: 'I have tried everything and have had no change in my condition, I don't know why I came, there is nothing to do.'

'Tell me, please, what is the problem,' I asked and she said: 'I keep falling at least once a week for the last seven years and it is lowering my confidence on the street and even at home. I can't go to the gym or do any other physical activity, and I am afraid it will last forever and I will be fat!'

She then continued, 'I was referred from a friend whom you helped but I am skeptical you will be able to "save" me. I have few expectations, so just do whatever you can.'

History-taking revealed that M. had no prior injuries or operations. The only problem she had had in the past was that as a newborn she had had full leg casts on both legs, toes to hips, due to pronounced internal rotation of the shins.

Methodology

As there were no clear signs on movement verification (MoVe), the treatment was based on the palpation. Given the history of leg casts as a newborn, palpation verification (PaVe) was carried out in all segments in the lower limb and also in the pelvis. In FM, asterisks are used to record pain on palpation (*), a palpable sensation of densification (*), and if any referred pain is elicited during palpation (*). It highlighted bilateral (bi) densifications, or alterations in the gliding of the deep fascia, in the centers of coordination (CC) on the frontal plane and to a lesser extent on the horizontal plane, with several points also referring pain along the limbs (***).

Palpation verification

Findings on initial palpation verification (PaVe) are as shown in Table 5.1.

Treatment

1st treatment: frontal plane (Table 5.2)

As I had no significant pre-treatment movement verifications to immediately verify the quality and accuracy of the treatment, I had to wait for the next session to evaluate the results.

CHAPTER 5

Table 5.1 Initial palpation verification						
Frontal plane	me-pe bi ***	la-pe bi**	me-ta bi**	me-ge bi***	me-cx bi**	la-pv bi***
Horizontal plane	ir-pe bi**	er-pv bi**				

Table 5.2 1st Treatment						
Points treated	me-pe bi	me-ta bi	me-ge bi	me-cx bi	la-pe bi	la-pv bi

Table 5.3 2nd Treatment				
Points treated	me-pe bi	me-ta bi	me-ge bi	me-cx bi
	la-pe bi	la-pv bi	me-pv	me-pv r

One week after the first treatment M. reported that there had already been a change, with much less falling and she was also feeling more secure on her feet.

2nd treatment (Table 5.3)

Given the progress made after the first treatment, the second treatment involved repetition of FM treatment on the above points on the frontal plane, all of which required less time to be cleared as compared to the first treatment; in addition, the me-pv anterior and posterior points were also treated (Table 5.3).

By the third FM treatment M. was really happy because during the 2 weeks between the second and the third session she had only had three falls. Treatment was completed on the frontal plane and balance exercises were added (Figure 5.1).

I needed to be sure of the outcome so I invited M. for a follow-up fourth session, which was planned for approximately 6 weeks after her very first treatment session. She reported that she had no longer had any falls, was completely satisfied and she said that her life had changed entirely.

The smile was now a part of M.'s life.

Considerations

This young woman's complaint had started 7 years before when she was 15 years of age. A recent systematic review (Fuglkjær et al. 2017) found that, in general population studies, the ankle, foot and knee were the most frequently reported anatomical complaint sites in children and adolescents. Together with the history of leg casts as a newborn that may have left some areas of fascial limitation, it was considered that development of the musculoskeletal system due to pubertal growth could have left her fascial tissue behind in terms of length, inducing the presenting symptoms. This may fall into the general category of what years ago used to be called 'growing pains.'

Case 2: severe sciatic-type pain in an elderly man

J. is an 88-year-old man who was brought to my clinic in a wheelchair. His condition was not an easy one. He had a strong tremor with atrophic muscles in his hands and especially in his legs, and he was unable to get up from the wheelchair unless he was helped.

J. had been healthy, exercising regularly and very active until he had a strong back pain episode with radiation to

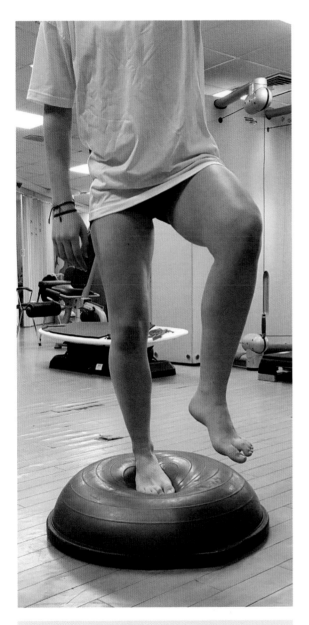

Figure 5.1
The use of BOSU® Balance Trainer as a type of pre-treatment and post-treatment movement verification can be helpful in cases of lower limb instability, such as in Case 1

his right leg, extending down to the lateral side of the right foot. This constant, debilitating pain was exacerbated by any change in position, such as turning in bed, and had constrained him to moving with a wheelchair. This had all started a month prior to coming to my clinic and the prolonged sitting was obviously not doing him any good. No X-rays had been taken at this stage and no other imaging was available. Asked about his past, J. reported that he had not had any operations. As a teenager, he had had only one fracture of his left tibia and fibula.

Methodology

Movement verification

Movement verification (MoVe) showed full range of motion (ROM) in the lumbar spine and the lower limbs but pain was felt with straight leg raise (SLR) at 60°.

Clearly, the entire MoVe could only be performed by means of passive moments and the pain was severe (***). When the MoVe is severely limited by pain, then palpation verification is the next step.

Palpation verification (Table 5.4)

Palpation verification (PaVe) of only the CCs did not offer any convincing signs of densification, although there were a few densified points on the sagittal plane; therefore, I also checked the centers of fusion (CF) in the foot (pe), ankle (ta), knee (ge), and hip (cx) segments. Because of the muscular atrophy, it was not easy to locate the CF points but I did find enough, in particular along the ante-latero (an-la) and ante-medio (an-me) diagonals. Findings on initial PaVe included the points recorded in Table 5.4.

Treatment

1st treatment (Table 5.5)

Treatment involved working on CFs along the ante-latero and ante-medio diagonals as well as a few CCs on the sagittal plane (Table 5.5).

Since it was very difficult for J. to change positions, the treatment took a very long time and I had to improvise a little, in terms of treatment positions, both for myself and the patient.

CHAPTER 5

Table 5.4 Initial palpation verification			
CCs	re-ta rt **	re-ge rt **	re-pv rt **
CFs	an-la-pe rt **	an-la-ta rt ***	an-la-cx rt ***
	an-me-pe rt **	an-me-ta rt ***	an-me-ge rt **

Table 5.5 1st Treatment						
CFs	an-la-pe rt	an-la-ta rt	an-la-cx rt	an-me-pe rt	an-me-ta rt	an-me-cx rt
CCs	re-ta rt	re-ge rt	re-pv rt			

2nd treatment

One week later, at the beginning of the second session, J. told me that because the pain had decreased, he had started to exercise a little in bed and also while sitting. It was amazing to see this trembling 88-year-old exercising with the determination of a young athlete but within his own capacity. The same points were treated again in this session, with the exception of an-me-cx, which was replaced by an-me-ge rt.

3rd–6th treatments

The third session was a surprise for me when J. came in walking on a walker, with his son just supervising him. The spark in J.'s eyes made it clear that change had happened – that spark was saying 'he is back'!

We had two more treatments after that just to make sure the pain did not return. Treatment proceeded on the ante-latero and ante-medio diagonals. By the fifth treatment, there was no pain on SLR on the right.

It was heartwarming for me to be able to help an 88-year-old man recover that big smile, which even the tremor could not prevent.

Considerations

Despite the patient's age and associated problems (tremor), pain resolved and function had been restored within just six treatments, the latter two being similar to merely control sessions to ensure the symptoms had not returned. The absence of imaging, as may often occur with direct access patients, should not necessarily be a deterrent for applying soft-tissue work judiciously. According to Weiner et al. (2006), biomechanical and soft tissue pathologies in older adults can be assessed reliably using a brief physical examination, saving unnecessary health care expenditure and patient suffering.

Case 3: runner's knee pain

A., a 30-year-old computer worker, called me over the phone and he had a lot of questions about the FM treatment and how it is different from other treatments that he had experienced in the last 18 months. A. lived in the countryside and he was an amateur runner. He used to run 50–60 kilometers a week and, when he decided to run a marathon for the first time, he had increased to 90 kilometers per week, and that was the beginning of his current injury or dysfunction.

When A. came to my clinic I saw he had a runner's body: slim and strong. However, his face disclosed his disappointment with his body.

The pain was on the lateral side of his left knee and, initially, it was 'bursting' after the eighth kilometer but now the pain (VRS 10/10) was occurring at the fourth kilometer. Since I am a triathlete myself, I know this type of pain and the intensity it can hit you with.

In the interview, A. told me that over the last 2 months he was also experiencing a milder, recurrent anterior pain in his right knee when going up stairs (in Stecco

Is this method magic? Certainly not. Three case reports

Eran Mangel

abbreviations: ge an rt 2m rec 2/10). He had had a severe left ankle sprain 2 years previously, a dislocation of his right shoulder 5 years previously, and a fracture to his right clavicle 8 years previously (in Stecco abbreviations: ta la rt 2y sprain; hu ir 5y lt disloc; sc an 8y lt fracture). This type of information allows the therapist to construct a timeline of previous injuries, traumas or events in order to elaborate a hypothesis.

Hypothesis

This combination of rather significant previous trauma presented me with a dilemma. Should I look for the cause of the present knee dysfunction in the same side foot or in the contralateral clavicle/shoulder? What brings more consequences: a severe sprain or a fracture followed by a dislocation? This was not easy. How do you explain to an athlete who almost lives 'in the web', and definitely works there, that the shoulder area could be responsible for his 'runner's knee'? Fortunately, he had tried everything before and nothing had helped. The answer was in the palpation verification (PaVe).

Methodology

Movement verification (MoVe)

As is often the case with athletes, clinical MoVes were not so significant (to reproduce the main symptoms I would have had to have him run 4 kilometers around my clinic!), therefore I moved directly on to palpation verification.

Palpation verification (PaVe)

In this first palpation verification (PaVe), I chose to palpate from the right upper quarter (scapula: sc) down to the left hip (coxa: cx). This PaVe highlighted numerous densified and painful CCs on the horizontal plane, also in the trunk segments between the shoulder and the hip (thorax: th, lumbi: lu, pelvis: pv).

Results from the initial PaVe are shown in Table 5.6.

Treatment

1st treatment: horizontal plane (Table 5.7)

2nd treatment

A week after the first treatment, A. reported that he had initially felt better for a few days, but then the symptoms returned again (+-). I repeated the first treatment again.

3rd treatment

Ten days after the second treatment, A. reported some improvement. Once again treatment addressed the horizontal plane (Table 5.8).

This third session was the game-changer and 2 days later he began running again.

I saw A. again for three sessions even though he was pain-free from the fifth session.

We had some ups and downs because he was eager to run as before, but eventually we came to an agreement

Table 5.6 Initial palpation verification				
irsc rt ***	er sc rt**	er th rt***	ir lu rt **	er lu lt**
er pv lt***	er cx lt ***	ir cx lt**	la cx lt**	

Table 5.7 1st Treatment						
ir-sc rt	ir-lu rt	ir-cx lt	er-sc rt	er-th rt	er-lu lt	er-pv lt

Table 5.8 3rd Treatment						
ir-sc rt	ir-th rt	ir-lu lt	ir-cx lt	er-sc rt	er-lu lt	er-cx lt

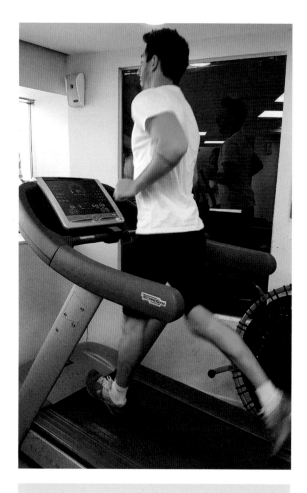

Figure 5.2
Post-treatment running training before returning to running outdoors

and he did what he was supposed to do by gradually increasing the length and the speed of his running (Figure 5.2), as suggested by Allen (2014) for gait retraining in long-distance runners.

Considerations

It is interesting to note that none of the CCs in the painful left knee segment (ge lt) required treatment at any time and that the game-changing treatment involved treatment of the left hip (er-cx lt). Furthermore, given that deep fascia is anatomically continuous with the paratenon that surround tendons (Stecco et al. 2014), manual therapy directed at fascia possibly influences the elastic properties of tendons, aiding stretch and recoil and the ability to store and return elastic strain energy during running (Alexander 2002).

Conclusion

For 25 years prior to entering into the world of the FM way of analysis, I treated thousands of people and always the thought was in my head, 'did I do enough?' Every physiotherapist has this phase in their professional life and the frustration is incessant. I am glad I was exposed to this new way of thinking and this effective method so I can help my patients in the best way possible.

Is this method magic? Certainly not. Three case reports

Eran Mangel

References

Alexander RM (2002) Tendon elasticity and muscle function. Comparative Biochemistry and Physiology Part A: Molecular and Integrative Physiology 133 (4) 1001–11.

Allen DJ (2014) Treatment of distal iliotibial band syndrome in a long-distance runner with gait re-training emphasizing step rate manipulation. International Journal of Sports Physical Therapy 9 (2) 222–31.

Branchini M, Lopopolo F, Andreoli E, Loreti I, Marchand AM and Stecco A (2016) Fascial Manipulation® for chronic aspecific low back pain: a single blinded randomized controlled trial. F1000 Research 4 1208.

Findley TW (2011) Fascia research from a clinician/scientist's perspective. International Journal of Therapeutic Massage and Bodywork 4 (4) 1–6.

Fuglkjær S, Dissing KB and Hestbæk L (2017) Prevalence and incidence of musculoskeletal extremity complaints in children and adolescents. A systematic review. BMC Musculoskeletal Disorders 18 (1) 418. doi:10.1186/s12891-017-1771-2.

Kalichman L, Lachman H and Freilich N (2016) Long-term impact of ankle sprains on postural control and fascial densification. Journal of Bodywork and Movement Therapies 20 (4) 914–19.

Pavan PG, Stecco A, Stern R and Stecco C (2014) Painful connection: Densification versus fibrosis of fascia. Current Pain and Headache Reports 18 (8) 441.

Picelli A, Ledro G, Turrina A, Stecco C, Santilli V and Smania N (2011) Effects of myofascial technique in patients with subacute whiplash associated disorders: A pilot study. European Journal of Physical and Rehabilitation Medicine 47 (4) 561–8.

Stecco C (2015) Functional atlas of the human fascial system. Edinburgh: Churchill Livingstone Elsevier

Stecco C, Cappellari A, Macchi V, Porzionato A, Morra A, Berizzi A and De Caro R (2014) The paratendineous tissues: an anatomical study of their role in the pathogenesis of tendinopathy. Surgical and Radiologic Anatomy 36 (6) 561–72. doi: 10.1007/s00276-013-1244-8.

Stecco L (2004) Fascial manipulation for musculoskeletal pain. Padua: Piccin.

Weiner DK, Sakamoto S, Perera S, Breuer P (2006) Chronic low back pain in older adults: Prevalence, reliability, and validity of physical examination findings. Journal of the American Geriatrics Society 54 (1) 11–20.

Section 2
Internal dysfunctions

The seven chapters in this section refer to the model developed by Luigi Stecco for the treatment of internal dysfunctions. Dysfunctions in this category are generally related to densifications in the superficial and/or internal fasciae, and their treatment aims to restore function within the autonomic nervous system, either by rebalancing tensile structures or by restoring fluidity within quadrants of the superficial fascia. As deep muscular fascia may also be involved in these dysfunctions, either as a primary cause or as a secondary consequence, some treatments may start with the musculoskeletal approach and then shift to the internal dysfunctions approach or vice versa. The points used in the treatment of internal dysfunctions are the same as those used for musculoskeletal dysfunctions but the association of points and the modality of treatment differs.

Tensional compensations from the musculoskeletal system to internal dysfunctions … or vice versa?

Andrea Pasini and Lorenzo Freschi, Italy

EDITOR'S COMMENT

This case report illustrates the complex relationship that appears to exist between musculoskeletal symptoms and internal dysfunctions. The two authors have studied directly with Luigi Stecco and are the first physiotherapists in the world to teach the practical applications of Fascial Manipulation for Internal Dysfunctions (FMID). Their expertise in this more recent therapeutic approach has contributed to spreading this knowledge internationally. Their case report is an analysis of the clinical reasoning process behind the treatment of chronic bilateral heel pain in a 43-year-old woman. Initially applying the musculoskeletal approach, only to find that results did not last more than a few days, more in-depth questioning leads them to apply the FMID approach, which proves to be considerably more effective. Furthermore, a post-treatment follow-up after 7 months reveals interesting developments related to altered internal structures.

Author's background

Andrea Pasini

My career in manual therapies started in 2001, working as a sports massage therapist with an amateur soccer team (Savignanese, Italy) while I completed my physiotherapy degree. After graduation from the Alma Mater Studiorum – University of Bologna, Italy, in 2003, I continued working with the soccer team but I also began working in private practice. The techniques I initially studied and applied include Global Postural Re-education method by Souchard, Bienfait's soft-tissue techniques, in particular pompage, and various forms of electrotherapy such as TENS, ultrasound, and laser therapy. I currently work in private practice and I teach Fascial Manipulation for Internal Dysfunctions (FMID).

Experience with Fascial Manipulation®– Stecco® method

When I started studying Fascial Manipulation®– Stecco® method (FM) in 2004, I was immediately impressed by two main aspects:

1. the reduction in the number of treatment sessions required to reach a more than satisfactory result

2. the possibility to achieve good results even in the acute phase.

FM sessions are carried out only once a week, whereas pompage, postural techniques, and electrotherapy require daily sessions for at least 10 sessions. Initially, I was dubious that weekly treatments could give results but the opposite actually occurred – results were much more evident than after daily sessions of pompage, postural techniques, and electrotherapy! This observation radically changed my practice. I started seeing more patients but for just a single weekly session each and generally discharging them from treatment much sooner, saving my patients both time and money. Furthermore, with acute conditions, I was previously limited to applying electrotherapy to decrease localized inflammation and pain, and then gradually introducing functional re-education. However, I would be forced to suspend the latter if pain flared up again. Instead, FM can be applied even in the acute phase because treatment is always applied at a distance from an inflamed area. Clearly, any contraindications or red flags need to be considered, but pain and inflammation are not contraindications to FM. While most methods concentrate on the symptomatic area, this approach taught me to look for the cause of the problem, which is often at a distance from the site of pain. In this way,

I was able to treat almost all acute patients, often with a significant decrease in symptoms in one or two sessions. Where necessary, I was subsequently able to treat the site of pain directly, respecting medical and evidence-based guidelines.

I observed that by using only therapies aimed at correcting postural tension without directly freeing the fascial densifications along the myofascial sequences, a stable improvement was not achieved. Therefore, I tried integrating the two approaches. Nevertheless, as suggested by Ćosić (Ćosić et al. 2014), I noted that as my experience in FM and my accuracy and efficiency in the manual technique improved, the postural work became progressively less essential.

Author's background

Lorenzo Freschi

Physiotherapist since 1994, I was team physiotherapist for the Cesena basketball team for 7 years. I have also worked in the public health sector for 20 years, including 15 years in a burn intensive care unit. I am currently in private practice. I started my FM studies in 1998, completing my Level I and II teacher training in musculoskeletal dysfunctions in 2012. I subsequently moved on to become a teacher of FMID, also known as Level III.

Experience with Fascial Manipulation®– Stecco® method

My first experience with FM was as a patient. I suffered from chronic low back pain that was rapidly resolved by this approach, giving me the impetus to study the method myself. Two key aspects of this method are:

1. its apparent efficacy and efficiency that, when the fascial component is preponderant, yield optimal results in a limited number of treatment sessions

2. the possibility to hypothesize and, subsequently, to distinguish the genesis of a fascial

dysfunction by means of an accurate interview that leads to the compilation of the method-specific assessment chart.

This approach generates a personalized application of FM, based on the patient's individual disturbances and aimed at the resolution of their problems without following any standardized protocols.

This way of reasoning falls into the scientific category of the 'health arts.' Analysis starts from the symptoms, the cause is hypothesized, the hypothesis is verified by means of movement and palpatory verifications and results are evaluated immediately after treatment and in subsequent follow-up sessions.

This approach stimulates therapists to develop an increasingly comprehensive interpretation of the physical, visceral, and psychogenic disturbances that manifest in each patient. Initially, it is necessary to break this approach into components (musculoskeletal versus visceral versus psychogenic) in order to analyze the way in which it functions. However, with practice, it is possible to select and often unite the different manual techniques included in FM in order to provide the answer to a specific distress.

In the near future, a further evolution of this method could lead to the interpretation of dysfunction as an expression of a global disturbance that, according to chronicity, spreads to the physical, visceral, and psychogenic spheres. We need to remind ourselves that we are merely the instrument or key that helps the patient to re-establish their own harmony and well-being.

CASE REPORT

Tensional compensations from the musculoskeletal system to internal dysfunctions ... or vice versa?

Tensional compensations from the musculoskeletal system to internal dysfunctions ... or vice versa?

Andrea Pasini and Lorenzo Freschi

This case was one of those 'milestone cases' that helped both of us in our initial stages of working with FMID to understand it better and to move forward with our clinical reasoning. It has a linear chronology and it illustrates how the fascia reorganizes the bodily functions for its own homeostasis and well-being.

Introduction

S. C., a 43-year-old woman, presented with bilateral calcaneal pain, on the right side more than the left, present for 5–6 months. Her work as a selector in a poultry breeding farm, necessitated standing for about 8 hours a day, but she was not required to lift any particularly heavy weights. She attended gym three times a week but was still marginally overweight (80 kg and 170 cm tall; body mass index: 28). Pain on the verbal rating scale (VRS) varied from 5/10 during the night to 9/10 in the morning on weight-bearing. Pain on weight-bearing was so intense that S. C. had been forced to modify her working position by sitting on a high stool. However, walking and standing were still very painful. In the first few months, when the pain was less, it was accompanied by a sensation of heavy legs that were at times also painfully swollen. Doppler ultrasonography of the lower limbs proved to be negative. X-rays of the feet highlighted significant heel spurs, distributed in the calcaneal and plantar regions, as well as around the Achilles tendon.

There was no previous history of tendinosis or trauma, fractures, or sprains, either in the ankle or in other regions. There was no reported concomitant pain, but previous pain included low back pain (LBP) in the paramedian sacral region that had started 8 years previously. This LBP was occasionally recurrent, lasting a few days but resolving quickly with a single dose of a common anti-inflammatory medicine. S. C. associated this sacral pain with work-related stress in the prolonged standing position. Gym work over the last 2–3 years had apparently reduced recurrences.

Questioned about internal organ dysfunctions, S. C. recently revealed that she had to take medicine for mild hypertension, which was of a possible genetic or familial origin given that both parents suffer from this complaint. She could not remember if hypertension had developed before or after the LBP.

Previous treatment, involving a series of laser therapy and ultrasound treatments directed to the painful heels, had yielded no results. Subsequent ultrasonography and magnetic resonance examinations of the Achilles tendon diagnosed bilateral enthesopathy and plantar fasciitis, treated with a second series of laser therapy and ultrasound treatments, anti-inflammatories and orthotics but without results. S. C. was then advised to try localized cortisone and lidocaine injections; however, she opted to try some FM treatments prior to proceeding with these injections.

Hypothesis

Following the anamnesis, a hypothesis was elaborated. Given the lack of previous trauma or musculoskeletal dysfunctions the hypothesis was divided between two options:

1. a musculoskeletal dysfunction due to work-related functional overuse of the lumbar (lu), pelvic (pv) and ankle (ta) regions. Different articles in literature associate postural changes, loading and heel pain (Cruz-Montecinos et al. 2015; Kirkpatrick et al. 2017)

2. due to hypertension, an internal dysfunction involving the circulatory apparatus (ACI) (Stecco L. & Stecco A. 2016). This dysfunction could have caused secondary tensional compensation in the musculoskeletal system.

Hence, in S. C.'s case, the direction of tensional compensations could have developed either in a somato-visceral or a visceral-somatic direction. Doubts remained concerning the chronological order of the LBP and the hypertension, and the latter could be familial. In addition, the patient had an occupation that put demands on her postural stability and, despite regular exercise, she was still rather overweight.

CHAPTER 6

Therefore, in order to proceed with movement and palpation verification, the first hypothesis of musculoskeletal dysfunction was chosen.

Methodology

Movement verification (MoVe)

Movement verification (MoVe) revealed an inability to weight-bear on her heels, with referred pain extending up the posterior leg. This referred pain could be due to an excessive stress on the crural and plantar fasciae. As these fasciae are in continuity (Stecco et al. 2013; Wilke et al. 2016), if one is too stiff it can pull on the other, resulting in referred pain.

Palpation verification (PaVe)

Palpation verification (PaVe) highlighted densified centers of coordination (CC) on several planes, the worst being the sagittal plane, followed by the horizontal plane. There were also densified centers of fusion (CF) on several diagonals, particularly in the ankle (ta) and knee (ge). All points in the foot (pes) were also painful and tense. Altered points in the ta and ge segments indicated two potentially altered diagonals, namely ante-medio and retro-latero, but no confirmation of either diagonal was found during specific palpation in the pe and pelvis (pv) segments.

1st treatment (Table 6.1)

Given the overall symptoms and signs, treatment was started from the sagittal plane.

The densified CCs of the myofascial units responsible for movement on the sagittal plane were treated in the knee (ge), ankles (ta), and feet (pe) (Figure 6.1).

Immediately after treatment, S. C. was able to walk without limping (VRS 4/10). Single leg weight-bearing was still painful but without referred pain.

Status after 1st treatment

After 1 week, S. C. reported that while the treated points had been sore to touch for a few days, the night after treatment was pain-free and the next morning she was able to weight-bear with less pain. The first 2 days posttreatment were mostly pain-free, except when ascending the stairs and pivoting on the right foot. However, from day 3 the situation slowly deteriorated, with the previous heel symptoms returning, although the referred leg pain was absent. Having clarified that no adverse events had occurred to produce this regression, S. C. was asked if any other symptoms had emerged after treatment. She reported having had an intense headache in the first 2 days, similar to but even stronger than what she normally experienced at the beginning of her menstrual cycle. She had taken pain medication to ease it.

Asked about any menstrual problems, such as rhythm, blood flow, or pain, she responded negatively. When questioned about any glandular problems related to the thyroid or liver, rather irritated at what she deemed inappropriate questioning she nevertheless recalled a mild hypothyroidism that did not require medication but was possibly the cause of a slower metabolism, which she associated with her difficulty in losing weight.

Insisting, we asked about any symptoms in the internal organs of the pelvic region, in particular, symptoms regarding the intestines, bladder, and reproductive organs. S. C. reported that she had an asymptomatic ovarian cyst of 3 centimeters on the right side, which had been monitored over the last 6 or 7 years.

Formulation of second hypothesis

This new information suggested that her heel pain could be related to the ovarian cyst in the pelvic region, which, together with the hypothyroidism and premenstrual headaches, indicated a possible dysfunction in the glandular sequence, in particular, of the endocrine apparatus (AEN) (Stecco L. & Stecco A. 2016).

Table 6.1					
Points treated	re-ta rt	an-ge rt	an-pe rt	re-ta lt	an-pe lt

Tensional compensations from the musculoskeletal system to internal dysfunctions ... or vice versa?

Andrea Pasini and Lorenzo Freschi

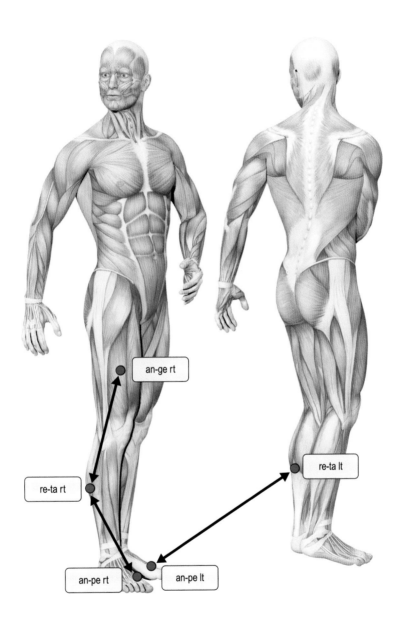

Figure 6.1
Illustration of densified centers of coordination of the myofascial units responsible for movement on the sagittal plane that were treated in the knee (ge), ankles (ta), and feet (pe) during the first treatment. On the right leg: antemotion-genu (an-ge rt), retromotion talus (re-ta rt), and antemotion-pes (an-pe rt), and on the left leg, retromotion-talus (re-ta lt) and antemotion-pes (an-pe lt). The black arrows indicate the lines of tension connecting the points

Therefore, the decision was taken to apply the FMID approach for the second treatment.

2nd palpation verification

With FMID, PaVe is initially directed at the anterior trunk wall. It highlighted two prevalent lines of tension (catenaries): anteroposterior (AP) and oblique (OB) lines. The second step of PaVe was the 'control catenaries' in the cervical (cl) and cephalic (cp) segments, which established that the anteroposterior (AP) catenaries, namely ante-medio and retro-medio, had the most important densifications. The third step of PaVe, directed at the 'distal tensors' in the lower limbs (ta and pe segments), once again highlighted densified CFs on the ante-medio and retro-medio catenaries.

While the vascular sequence is generally associated with the AP catenaries and the glandular sequence with the oblique (OB) catenaries (intrarotation and extrarotation), in this particular case, given that the overall association of points was scattered in numerous segments, including the pelvis, lower limbs, head, neck, and upper limbs, the hypothesis of an AEN dysfunction was confirmed.

2nd treatment (Figure 6.2; Table 6.2)

After treatment of the most painful and densified points in the retro-medio and ante-medio catenaries and the relative associated points (retro points), as well as distal tensors in the ankle segment (re-me-ta bi), the movement verification was asymptomatic, as it was after the first session.

Results

One week after the second treatment, S. C. reported, via telephone, that all symptoms had completely disappeared. The patient was asked to refer back after the ultrasonography examination of the ovarian cyst,

programmed for 6 months later. In effect, 7 months later the patient reported that she had not had any heel pain and that the ultrasonography had confirmed that the ovarian cyst had been completely absorbed.

Discussion

This case report highlights the analytical process required to elaborate a hypothesis that considers the entire body. It also presents some interesting aspects of the interaction of the internal organs with the musculoskeletal system and how the distribution of tension can occur from the internal organs towards the periphery (visceral-somatic).

FMID treatment, indeed FM treatment in general, is always preceded by the elaboration of a hypothesis. First, the indecision regarding the initial hypothesis (musculoskeletal versus internal dysfunctions) was related to the fact that there was not a precise cause of pain. Usually in FM, and even in FMID, we look for a previous disorder that can generate a chain of tensional compensations. A previous disorder can be a trauma, surgery, or an internal dysfunction. In this case, there was no important previous problem or trauma in the musculoskeletal system, which led us to formulate the second hypothesis about an internal dysfunction. The symptoms of swollen legs and mild hypertension could be related to a dysfunction of the circulatory apparatus but:

1. the first symptom could be also related to excessive tightness in the muscular fascia of the inferior limbs

2. the second symptom appeared to be less important and possibly genetic.

Furthermore, the circulatory apparatus is strictly connected with the lower limb muscular fasciae and the posterior trunk fasciae. The fascia of the large abdominal

Table 6.2				
Points treated	re-ta bi	re-me-ta bi	re-me pv bi	an-me-pv 2 rt
	an-me-lu 2 rt	an-me-th 2 lt	an-me-cl rt	re-cl lt

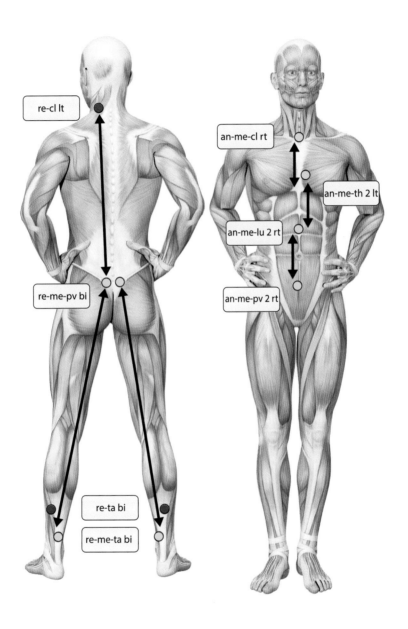

Figure 6.2

Illustration of the centers of coordination and fusion that were treated during the second treatment. In the neck, retromotion collum on the left (re-cl lt) and ante-medio collum on the right (an-me-cl rt); in the thorax, ante-medio thorax on the left (an-me-th lt); in the lumbar segment, ante-medio lumbi 2 on the right (an-me-lu 2 rt); in the pelvis, retro-medio pelvis bilaterally (re-me-pv bi) and ante-medio pelvis 2 on the right (an-me-pv 2 rt); in the talus, retromotion talus bilaterally (re-ta bi) and retro-medio talus bilaterally (re-me-ta bi). The black arrows indicate the lines of tension connecting the points vessels (aorta, vena cava) and that of the kidneys (renal fascia, or Gerota's fascia) are in continuity with the pre-vertebral fascia and the thoracolumbar fascia (Stecco L. & Stecco A. 2016). This explains how the minor circulatory apparatus dysfunction (mild hypertension) could have developed secondarily to rigidity in the posterior trunk fasciae, which might also relate to the occasional bouts of LBP.

Instead, the alternative or purely musculoskeletal hypothesis found some support in the X-ray signs (heel spurs) and the prolonged standing position required for work. Hypotheses are not binding but they do orientate the type of palpation verification that is carried out. Faced with a decision, the therapist makes a therapeutic choice based on the best available information. However, it is also important to be able to analyze why a particular treatment gives only temporary relief and, based on the outcome, how to improve results at the following session. In our practice, supported also by literature (Vulcano et al. 2014; Ramin et al. 2016), it happens quite frequently that we have heel pain in patients without any significant findings in the examinations, or conversely, patients with no heel pain in the presence of heel spurs.

Secondly, the fact that the patient reported a definite improvement in symptoms in the distal segment (pe) after the first treatment but also the appearance of an intense headache (cp) indicated that fascial tension was released in the lower limbs but had increased in the upper part of the body, specifically towards the head. According to the FMID biomechanical model, the extremities (ankles/feet, wrists/hands, and head) are the areas in which the body can spread fascial tension due to an internal dysfunction: in other words from the contents (internal organs) to the container (trunk wall), and from the trunk to the extremities. Quite often the patient's symptoms are in the extremities. Furthermore, the patient described this headache as similar to her 'usual' premenstrual headache, which generated the hypothesis of an endocrine apparatus (AEN) involvement (Kannan & Claydon 2014).

According to the model applied in FMID, the AEN is part of the glandular sequence and, when dysfunctional, it is common to find densifications scattered in a number of extremities (head, feet/lower leg, and hands/forearms) (Stecco et al. 2013). This hypothesis of an endocrine dysfunction was initially reinforced by the presence of a mild hypothyroidism, and further so with the revelation of an ovarian cyst. It is important to underline here that we address dysfunctions and not internal organ pathologies. In other words, we take into consideration areas where there are minor disturbances and where something requires monitoring but without pathological characteristics or an established diagnosis of pathology.

Thirdly, the second treatment session was orientated toward an FMID approach thanks to our rather tenacious questioning about symptoms in the pelvic internal organs, in particular regarding the intestines, bladder, and reproductive organs. The choice of targeting the pelvic region was related to the fact that the paramedian sacral region, where there was a history of LBP, lies between the presenting problem (heel pain) and the compensating disturbance (headache) (Torstensson et al. 2015). In all fascial dysfunctions, whether muscular or internal fasciae are involved, or a combination of both, the distribution of compensatory tension is not casual but follows predictable fascial connections.

In this particular case, the questioning was necessary in order to be able to understand whether the presenting dysfunctions were all connected with the glandular sequence or if other internal sequences could have been involved. S. C. acknowledged having an ovarian cyst of 3 centimeters diameter that had been regularly monitored by her gynecologist over the last 6 or 7 years. This new information shifted the hypothesis in a different direction. The heel pain could be related to, if not dependent upon, tension caused by the ovarian cyst that was present in the pelvic segment. At the initial data collection, the patient had not even mentioned this cyst because it was asymptomatic.

Nevertheless, in FMID it is known that even minor cyst formations in the pelvis can potentially be the source of tension that extends down the lower limbs.

The presence of the ovarian cyst, together with the mild hypothyroidism and the premenstrual headaches, directed the hypothesis towards the glandular sequence, in particular the endocrine apparatus, hence justifying the FMID approach in the second treatment.

Interestingly, at the next ultrasonography examination of the pelvic region, 6 months after the second FM treatment, it was found that the ovarian cyst had been completely reabsorbed. As confirmed by the gynecologist, this can happen, even though, according to the patient, the specialist was rather surprised. The fact that the heel pain had also completely disappeared does give food for thought. In effect, as therapists, we should also be asking 'what happened to the heel spurs?' (Williams et al. 1987).

Conclusion

This case report underlines how tensional compensation can develop in an attempt to protect the internal organs to the detriment of the musculoskeletal system, and how tension from internal organs may be transmitted towards the extremities in an attempt to recreate tensional harmony. This tensional balance is the basis for the correct functioning of the autonomic ganglia that control the smooth muscles of the viscera, vessels, and some glands (Stecco L. & Stecco C. 2014).

Furthermore, it demonstrates how the presenting symptom does not necessarily indicate the region or the cause of the dysfunction. With increasing experience and knowledge of fascial anatomy, the dichotomy of musculoskeletal and internal dysfunctions, which is quite difficult to understand in the beginning, becomes a mere didactical debate. The completeness and complexity of the FM method can only be mastered with dedication and passion for anatomy and physiology, together with a constant clinical practice.

To quote the founder of this method, Luigi Stecco: 'you find what you look for but you look for what you know,' from which stems this method's logo 'Manus sapiens potens est' ('a knowledgeable hand is powerful'), two principles that summarize the effort and dedication of the man who has developed this therapeutic approach.

CHAPTER 6

References

Ćosić V, Day JA, Iogna Prat P and Stecco A (2014) Fascial manipulation method applied to pubescent postural hyperkyphosis: A pilot study. Journal of Bodywork and Movement Therapies 18 (4) 608–15. doi: 10.1016/j.jbmt.2013.12.011.

Cruz-Montecinos C, González Blanche A, López Sánchez D, Cerda M, Sanzana-Cuche R and Cuesta-Vargas A (2015) In vivo relationship between pelvis motion and deep fascia displacement of the medial gastrocnemius: Anatomical and functional implications. Journal of Anatomy 227 (5) 665–72. doi: 10.1111/joa.12370.

Kannan P and Claydon LS (2014) Some physiotherapy treatments may relieve menstrual pain in women with primary dysmenorrhea: A systematic review. Journal of Physiotherapy 60 (1) 13–21.

Kirkpatrick J, Yassaie O and Mirjalili SA (2017) The plantar calcaneal spur: A review of anatomy, histology, etiology and key associations. Journal of Anatomy 230 (6) 743–51. doi: 10.1111/joa.12607.

Ramin A, Macchi V, Porzionato A, De Caro R and Stecco C (2016) Fascial continuity of the pelvic floor with the abdominal and lumbar region. Pelviperineology 35 3–6.

Stecco C, Corradin M, Macchi V, Morra A, Porzionato A, Biz C and De Caro R (2013) Plantar fascia anatomy and its relationship with Achilles tendon and paratenon. Journal of Anatomy 223 (6) 665–76. doi:10.1111/joa.12111.

Stecco L and Stecco A (2016) Fascial manipulation for internal dysfunctions: Practical part. Padua: Piccin, pp 151, 159.

Stecco L and Stecco C (2014) Fascial manipulation for internal dysfunctions. Padua: Piccin.

Torstensson T, Butler S, Lindgren A, Peterson M, Eriksson M and Kristiansson P (2015) Referred pain patterns provoked on intra-pelvic structures among women with and without chronic pelvic pain: A descriptive study. PLoS One 10 (3). doi:10.1371/journal.pone.0119542.

Vulcano E, Mani SB, Do H, Bohne WH and Ellis SJ (2014) Association of Achilles tendinopathy and plantar spurs. Orthopedics 37 (10) 897–901.

Wilke J, Engeroff T, Nürnberger F, Vogt L and Banzer W (2016) Anatomical study of the morphological continuity between iliotibial tract and the fibularis longus fascia. Surgical and Radiologic Anatomy 38 (3) 349–52. doi: 10.1007/s00276-015-1585-6.

Williams PL, Smibert JG, Cox R, Mitchell R, Klenerman L (1987) Imaging study of the painful heel syndrome. Foot and Ankle 7 (6) 345–9.

Treatment for chronic neck pain post motor vehicle accident

Cheryl Megalos, Canada

EDITOR'S COMMENT

Many people live with chronic pain long after a motor vehicle accident that they have luckily survived leaves them with ongoing problems. Here the author presents a case report of a 32-year-old administrative worker who suffered chronic neck pain and headaches for more than 2 years after the vehicle that she was driving was hit by another car. Symptoms resolved within just three sessions, bringing lasting relief to a long-standing problem. A participant of the first English course of Fascial Manipulation® held in Italy in 2010, the author introduces her personal manner of recording faulty movement patterns when first assessing a patient. She discusses how treatment can evolve from an initial musculoskeletal approach to an internal dysfunctions approach, as in this case report. Treatment cannot be relegated to a series of protocols. It is based on a combination of the patient's individual symptoms and what the therapist perceives as being densified or altered. As fascial layers are restored to normal gliding, underlying densifications can emerge, demanding dynamic adaptation of treatment from one session to the next.

Author's background

After graduating from the University of British Columbia with a Bachelor of Science degree in 1994, I initially worked as a physiotherapist in a vocational setting with an orthopedic caseload, then in a manual therapy-based clinic from 1996 to the present day. I currently work as a manual physiotherapist in a busy orthopedic clinic in Vancouver (BC), Canada, focusing on the treatment of clients with chronic pain, myofascial disturbances, post-surgical care, such as after mastectomy surgery, as well as referrals from colleagues treating hand injuries and orofacial dysfunction. My postgraduate studies include the Canadian Academy of Manipulative Physiotherapy coursework, as well as certification in intramuscular stimulation (IMS) in 2007. I am a licensed physical therapist in the province of British Columbia, Canada, and the state of Hawaii, USA.

Introduction

As a physiotherapist working in a busy practice I am generally exposed to chronic conditions in an orthopedic setting. While I do collaborate with other colleagues, such as Certified Hand Therapists and clinicians who focus on temporomandibular joint pain, my clients include a variety of conditions and complex individual cases. With an education centered on an orthopedic and a joint-based school of thought, after completing courses with the Canadian Academy of Manipulative Physical Therapists, the focus of my practice was high-velocity thrust techniques of peripheral and spinal joints, exercises to work on muscular control of movement, and proper biomechanical analysis. This approach gave some good results but, after years of utilizing these techniques, I found that often the symptoms would recur. My instructors had always emphasized that a joint should not need to be manipulated multiple times; instead, some other force was likely in play, restricting the normalization of joint glide.

A needling technique, intramuscular stimulation (IMS), was another option to work on both the muscle and the nerves that also affect joints. The theory for this method considers addressing myofascial pain derived from a neuropathic pain model. I began to use dry needling as a modality after studying with Dr Chan Gunn. An improvement of joint mobility appeared to result, with less need to mobilize or manipulate joints. However, there were still individuals with recurrent symptoms. There was also a population that could not (or did not want to) be treated with needles. With these individuals, a soft tissue approach was employed in an attempt to have the same effect as with needles. I found 'neural tension' tests could be altered in the upper limb by only treating the thorax, but since I was not actually affecting deep muscle, as with the needle, it was unclear to me how this was occurring.

The experience of piercing a needle through fascia in different areas of the body, such as the thoracolumbar fascia and the thigh, also raised some questions about the structures below the skin and within the muscle. One could feel the needle pierce through thick distinguishing layers of tissue in some individuals, but not with others. As well, the feeling of lack of softness to some of the tissue being needled gave me pause for thought. For example, one could not get a needle into such tissue without guidance, as it felt more like trying to pierce into a solid structure, like wood, rather than a soft contractile tissue. What could be the reason for this?

For all these reasons I began to search out knowledge about fascia. My first course was in John Barnes's *Myofascial Release* approach (Barnes 1990). Unfortunately, there appeared to be a lack of research-based material being taught and, upon application of these techniques, I had limited and short-lived success. I then began to study Thomas Myers's *Anatomy Trains* text (Myers 2009), which gave me interesting information that I later found paralleled in other fascial researchers' work.

Inspired to attend the 2nd Fascial Research Congress in Amsterdam in 2009, I pored over the many options for workshops and keynote lectures, and Fascial Manipulation® by Luigi Stecco came to my attention. This is when I became aware of an upcoming Fascial Manipulation® (FM) course in Italy, the first course being offered in English (2010). After pondering the dilemma of having to travel to Italy, one of my favorite places in the world I might add, I decided to have a go at it! I prepared for the course by reading Luigi Stecco's Fascial Manipulation® text (2004), covering the theory of this technique and its anatomical and physiological basis. With the help of this book I plunged into my investigation of fascia, a new topic as a treatment focus for my education to date.

Experience with Fascial Manipulation®–Stecco® method

That first Fascial Manipulation®–Stecco® method (FM) course held in Italy was well organized and explored a new possibility of looking at the musculoskeletal system as put forth by the work of physiotherapist Luigi Stecco. It proposed a new biomechanical model to consider, once fascia was included with muscle, nerve, vascularity, joint, tendon and so forth. It suggested that fascia had malleability, particularly within the loose connective tissue component (Stecco A. et al. 2016), and that restriction in the fascia could be the source of long-term problems suffered by many people. However, this aspect was not being addressed by the current physiotherapy models of assessment and treatment. This was astounding! Most of all, when observing a treatment, to see that after manipulation of only a few carefully chosen points, which were often away from the area of reported pain, there can be a significant change, both objectively and subjectively, opened the way to new clinical reasoning options.

Since the introduction of FM to my practice, when someone reports a musculoskeletal problem, I no longer consider just the presenting complaint. Instead, in reference to the Stecco model (Stecco L. & Stecco C. 2009), a comprehensive history compilation allows a better understanding of how the problem evolves. Prior to this, insidious onset was a frequent comment, and it was simply accepted, both by my patient and myself! Now I ensure the symptoms and the person's history make sense prior to commencing the objective assessment and this continues throughout, prior to, and during the treatment. The satisfaction of having individuals improve, especially those who have had little success with other treatments, aimed at the nerve, muscle, and joint, has given me the impetus to pursue further studies regarding the fascial system.

Currently, this method is the mainstay of my practice. It allows me to analyze the body in such a way as to consider the tensional compensations creating changes in the fascial tissue throughout the body. Starting with this, many of the problems with recruitment of muscle and the elongation of tissue to allow improvement of range of motion (ROM) can be resolved. Fascia, a tissue which is highly innervated with proprioceptive organs, such as the Ruffini and Paccini corpuscles, as well as free nerve endings (Stecco C. et al. 2008; Tesarz et al. 2011), can affect the musculoskeletal system's response to stress and strain. Another important discovery in research is that the muscle spindle, an important stretch sensor that regulates recruitment of the alpha motor neuron, is very intimate with the fascial system, including the deep fascia, the epimysium, perimysium, and even the delicate endomysium (Stecco C. et al. 2007). If the muscle spindle is unable to respond due to an alteration in the mobility of the tissue, then ROM, muscle recruitment and, therefore, strength and proprioception can be affected. This can explain why after carefully instructing patients how to carry out, for example, core exercises, they cannot achieve the desired results, despite their compliance and dedication. After restoring the ability for the sensors within the fascia to transmit normal afferent information, rehabilitation can then include exercise to improve motor recruitment and movement of the body, thereby avoiding a recurrence of symptoms with the same inappropriate movements.

CASE REPORT

Treatment of chronic neck pain post motor vehicle accident

Introduction

G. is a 35-year-old woman who presented with lateral neck pain, more notable on her right side than on her left, together with significant tenderness in the antero-lateral cervical area. Associated lateral-sided headaches were also reported when neck symptoms worsened, many times a week. These symptoms are related to a motor vehicle accident that occurred 2.5 years prior to her presentation, when she was hit on the passenger side of the vehicle that she was driving. Two days after the accident she recalled having had cramps in her right calf, and pain in the left side of her neck, followed by pain in the right side. She also reported experiencing a problem with swallowing 6 months prior to the assessment (2 years after the injury), as well as dry eyes and numbness in the fourth and fifth digits on her left hand. Investigations included X-rays, magnetic resonance imaging, and electromyography, all of which were said to be negative, as per the referring physiatrist. Previous treatments, such as physiotherapy and massage therapy, were said to have had no lasting effect on her symptoms.

At the time of assessment, G. reported her neck symptoms being notably aggravated by ironing, mowing the lawn and postures at her job as an administrator.

Hypothesis

Given that G. had already undergone treatment with no relief of her pain, and had symptoms such as dry eyes, difficulty swallowing, and numbness in the left hand that, within the context of the Stecco biomechanical model, could be associated with the frontal plane, I hypothesized that working with the fascial system by addressing this structure would be very appropriate. In particular, symptoms were indicating involvement along the mediomotion myofascial sequence (see Discussion). Another hypothesis could have been dysfunction within the vascular sequence, which is part of the Fascial Manipulation for Internal Dysfunctions (FMID) model and includes the anteromedial and retromedial catenaries. This analysis of presenting signs and symptoms can always suggest a hypothesis, but it is never conclusive (as the first treatment demonstrates in this case). It has to be verified by an objective examination consisting of movement and palpatory tests. Nevertheless, by considering the patient's symptoms, history, and presenting signs within the context of Stecco's interpretation of the fascial system, it does help me to decide which body segments I examine with movement verification, which is the first part of the objective assessment used in FM.

Methodology

Movement verification (MoVe)

As G. appeared to be quite guarded with movements of her neck, in particular, I chose to examine the movements of the neck (collum: cl) and scapular segments (sc). In FM, asterisks are used to indicate pain, limited range of movement (ROM), or weakness. On my assessment charts, I also like to specify which of these elements was faulty and if other signs, such as fear or apprehension, are apparent. I do this by assigning a number to each element (1-restricted ROM, 2-apprehension, 3-pain with 'place and hold'). Therefore, I can record the results of the MoVe as in Table 7.1 (see explanation beneath each faulty movement).

Palpation verification (PaVe)

The cl segment was palpated first, followed by the right ankle segment (talus: ta). The latter segment was chosen because I was curious about the cramping that G. remembered feeling the day after her accident. Also, on observation, G. demonstrated varicosities into the left calf and posterior thigh and, when positioned in prone, I noted that her left foot and ankle were positioned so that the hindfoot was inverted when compared to the right (Figure 7.1).

In FM, asterisks are used once again to record pain on palpation, the therapist's perception of densification, and if any referred pain is elicited. Palpation verification revealed pain and densification in the centers of coordination (CC) as reported in Table 7.2.

1st treatment: horizontal plane

I chose to treat the horizontal plane (ir/er) since this was where the most significant densifications were evident.

Also, headaches running from the collum posteriorly and up to behind and above the ear into the cranial deep fascia can be associated with the horizontal plane. Therefore, these associations could possibly explain her headaches, which had a similar pattern (Table 7.3).

It is interesting to note here how treatment on one plane (horizontal) changed movements also on the frontal and sagittal planes, which is a common occurrence with this type of fascial work.

2nd session: 1 week later

When G. returned after 1 week she reported that 1 hour after the first treatment her retro-orbital headache had worsened for a short time, then pain referred also to the right side of her neck (cl rt) but, since then, she had not had any headaches.

PaVe was then extended to other segments – scapula, lumbar and thorax. Interestingly, there were now dominating signs of densification on the sagittal plane and some centers of fusion (CF) were also painful and densified.

2nd treatment: sagittal plane, with the addition of three CFs

I chose to change to the sagittal plane for a few reasons. My initial hypothesis was still valid regarding the symptoms, so with palpation of the extremities and torso, findings were noted along the midline, which is associated with the vascular sequence (Figure 7.2; Table 7.4).

Table 7.1 Movement verification

MoVe	la-cl bi* 1	re-cl** 2	an-cl*** 3	me-sc rt ***
Explanation of findings	Lateral flexion of the neck was restricted in ROM bilaterally	Apprehension limited her neck flexion (50%)	Pain with place and hold with head (supine)	Weakness of shoulder adduction from 120°
MoVe	la-sc-lt***	er-sc rt**	re-sc pain=>cu***	
Explanation of findings	Weakness of shoulder abduction from 120°	Restriction of right cervical rotation 50%	Resisted right scapular retraction referred pain to the elbow	

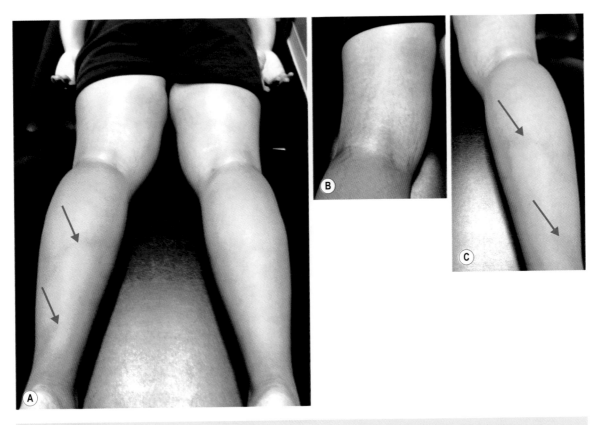

Figure 7.1
To demonstrate the veins on left leg, posteriorly, on the thigh and lower leg. Note also the internal rotation of hip and inverted hind foot on the left

Table 7.2 Initial palpation verification				
er-cl rt***	er-sc lt**	la-cl rt**	ir-cl rt**	ir-ta rt***

Table 7.3 1st Treatment				
Points treated	er-sc lt	er-th rt	er-th lt	ir-ta rt
MoVe improved after treatment	la-cl bi	re-sc	me-sc rt	

Table 7.4 2nd Treatment					
Points treated	re-me-cl lt	re-cl lt	re-sc lt	an-cl lt	me-cl
	an-me-sc 2 rt	re-me-th1 rt	an-cp1 lt	me-cp1 lt	

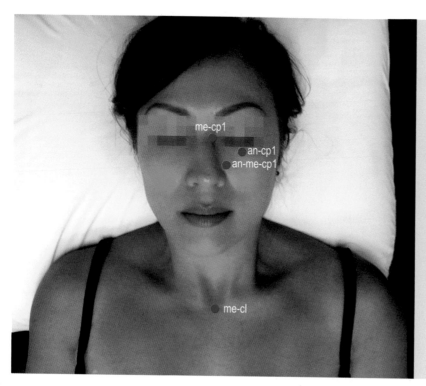

me-cp1
an-cp1
an-me-cp1

me-cl

Figure 7.2
One can often find alterations in the facial fascia at the medial canthus associated with dry eyes: center of coordination (CC) of medio-caput 1 on the left (me-cp1 lt). In particular, with this patient, the CC of ante-caput 1 on the left (an-cp1 lt) was also affected. Both points are connected with the center of fusion (CF) of ante-medio-caput 1 (an-me-cp1). Note also location of the CC of medio-collum (me-cl)

3rd session: 1 week later

G. reported that she had not had any headaches, but she had some pain alternating from rt to lt in the cervical area. Her reported difficulty with swallowing was not noticeably present nor could she recall having any difficulties during the last week. She also remembered that she had had a sprained ankle when she was younger (she was unsure which ankle it had been) but had forgotten about this during the initial anamnesis.

3rd treatment: FMID (Table 7.5)

Given that the possibly unresolved injury in her ankle that she had more recently recalled could be a factor contributing to her distal symptoms, treatment of the retro-medio CFs in the lower extremity and pelvis addressed the symptoms into her calves and the cramping at night. When utilizing the FMID approach of the Stecco method, it considers treating into the distal tensors of the extremities, as well as the head and neck, to help with symptoms that may be affecting the trunk. The pelvic and shoulder girdles are also important areas to assess and treat as part of FMID, as was done in this treatment, which included the CFs of re-me-cx bilaterally (Figures 7.4, 7.5), as well as, an-me-sc and re-me-sc.

After this treatment, there was a definite improvement in cl ROM in all directions as well as neck flexion strength (an-cl).

Results

After three treatments of FM, the patient demonstrated full cervical ROM, neck flexor strength, abolishment of

Table 7.5 3rd Treatment				
Points treated	re-me-ta 1 lt	me-ge lt	re-me-cx lt	re-me-cx rt
	re-me-sc lt	me-sc lt	me-lu 2 (Figure 7.3)	

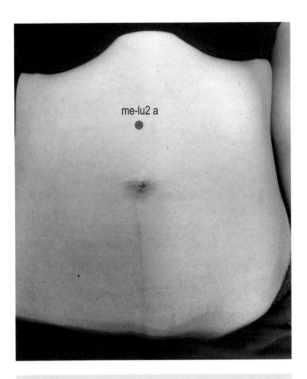

me-lu2 a

Figure 7.3
The patient mostly had findings down the linea alba and the spinous processes of her spine (centers of coordination of the mediomotion sequence) or just lateral to both linea alba and spine (centers of fusion of ante-medio and retro-medio). Here the CC of medio-lumbi 2 is illustrated

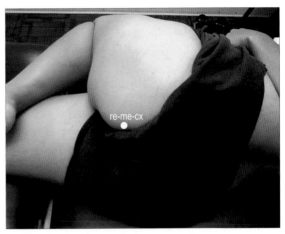

re-me-cx

Figure 7.4
Location of retro-medio-coxa (re-me-cx) over the pubococcygeal fascia, patient in side-lying

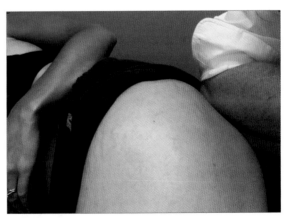

Figure 7.5
Position of therapist at the sacrum to access retro-medio-coxa most effectively, given the amount of tissue in this area

headaches and a significant reduction in neck pain. G. also reported that the dryness she experienced in her eyes had resolved. Reduction in calf cramping was noted but further work on proper postural hygiene and activation of hip muscles was needed. Ergonomic considerations, such as the fact she worked an administrative job in what she described as a 'closet space,' were also addressed to aid in recovery.

Discussion

When considering the focus of treatment, it seemed that G. had specific areas where the symptoms had settled and had not resolved, with the focus on the neck area in particular. Tensional compensations within fascia can

be experienced along a plane or can be associated with internal dysfunctions. These will not respond to treatment if you do not address other areas that could be implicated. The frontal plane includes the lateromotion and mediomotion sequences of the limbs and trunk. In particular, the mediomotion line of the trunk includes,

CHAPTER 7

anteriorly, the cervical linea alba, the pectoralis fascia that crosses over the sternum, and the linea alba in the abdomen and, posteriorly, over the spinous processes (crossover points), or namely the ligamentum nuchae, the supraspinous and interspinous ligaments of the thorax, the lumbar interspinous ligaments and over the raphe of the pubococcygeus fascia between the sacrum and the coccyx (Stecco L. 2004). These myofascial sequences can also be implicated in certain internal dysfunctions such as reported here. For example, dry eyes, which can be associated with the me-cp 1 CC; leg cramps with the CCs of me-lu, me-pv and me-cx, extending down to me-pe (Stecco L. 2004); problems with swallowing can be associated with densifications in me-cl (Stecco L. & Stecco C. 2013). In particular, the medial line can be associated with vascular issues, and this individual had varicosities in her legs, specifically on the left side (Stecco L. & Stecco C. 2013).

Previous to my discovery of the wide-ranging effects of FM, with its potential to influence and modify the extra-cellular component of the deep fascia (Pavan et al. 2014), and its implementation into my practice, I would not have considered that I could have had any effect on the swallowing, or the dry eyes (I likely would have scratched my head and disregarded both, being unable to treat them). Also, I would probably have only considered discussing the use of compression stockings for her varicosities as a way of advising her. Likely, I would have been very frustrated and puzzled as to why her neck symptoms did not respond to work around the spine. Currently, if I hear that an area has been treated directly and it has not given any lasting resolution, I immediately consider that it is not likely to be as straightforward as addressing the area of pain, solely.

By applying the Stecco model and employing the knowledge I now have about fascial connections, considering the location of symptoms certainly aided me in my clinical reasoning. However, with G., treating her mediomotion and/or vascular sequence gave a longer lasting effect to her chronic neck symptoms and calf cramps than treating the local area alone. When G. was first assessed for alteration in her fascial gliding,

densification indicated that the horizontal plane was more affected. However, the first treatment, which was directed to this plane, did not resolve the symptoms in her neck and the leg cramping completely. Palpation of the head and neck, the trunk and the extremities can prove to be extremely useful, as in this case, because it can highlight a certain plane or sequence which can then be investigated for involvement. There had been some stiffness in the me-cp1 rt when reviewed but it was not as involved initially. What can be interesting with FM is that ongoing assessment can show a resolution in densification and an apparent shifting of densities to other CCs or CFs after treatment, as noted when G. returned for the second treatment. It allows for a change in one's working hypothesis and, subsequently, the treatment approach. In this particular case, it moved from an initial musculoskeletal approach to one considering the likely vascular component. When G. returned for a subsequent treatment session several months later, she reported a cramping into her bladder, considered by Stecco as being part of the vascular sequence. This was then resolved with treatment of the medial ankle, coccygeal fascia, linea alba and supraspinous ligamentous areas, which are all fascial tissues typically implicated with the vascular sequence in Stecco's FMID model.

As a general follow-up for this chapter, 1 year after treatment commenced, G. reports that she occasionally feels sore over the right scapular ridge, and cramps in her calves can still occur after sitting for long periods. However, she notices that things settle quickly if she is able to do recruitment exercises for her trunk, shoulders, and hips. She has had no return of bladder cramping, headaches, dry eyes (apart from wearing contact lenses for an extended time), or any dysphagia.

Conclusion

This case study is merely one example of some very interesting results of clients presenting with chronic symptoms that were non-responsive to traditional treatments, such as articular mobilizations, muscular hands-on treatment and exercises, performed by other well-qualified therapists. What is especially outstanding to me is that by improving the gliding of the loose connective tissue within deep fascia, which few therapists are even aware of being able to effect, we can make immediate and lasting changes. As with G., some training may be needed to ensure the individual maintains deep fascia gliding and the patency of their fascial system while still managing the daily demands in their life, as pertains to our focus as physiotherapists. In addition, taking into account other complaints, such as cramping, dry eyes, and swallowing difficulties, can lead to a treatment direction, not to mention the ability to help the person with internal dysfunctions, which previously were not symptoms I thought I could affect. The Stecco method has given me more insight and clinical reasoning skills to guide my assessment and treatment, providing me with more satisfying and successful results.

References

Barnes JF (1990) Myofascial release: The search for excellence. USA: Rehabilitation Services Inc.

Myers TW (2009) Anatomy trains: Myofascial meridians for manual and movement therapists. Edinburgh: Churchill Livingstone, Elsevier.

Pavan PG, Stecco A, Stern R and Stecco C (2014) Painful connections: Densification versus fibrosis of fascia. Current Pain and Headache Reports 18 (8) 441.

Stecco A, Stern R, Fantoni I, De Caro R and Stecco C (2016) Fascial disorders: Implications for treatment. PM & R 8 (2) 161–8.

Stecco C, Gagey O, Belloni A, Pozzuoli A, Porzionato A, Macchi V, Aldegheri R, De Caro R and Delmas V (2007) Anatomy of the deep fascia of the upper limb. Second part: Study of innervation. Morphologie 91 (292) 38–43.

Stecco C, Porzionato A, Lancerotto L, Stecco A, Macchi V, Day JA and De Caro R (2008) Histological study of the deep fasciae of the limbs. Journal of Bodywork and Movement Therapies 12 (3) 225–30.

Stecco L (2004) Fascial manipulation for musculoskeletal pain. Padua: Piccin.

Stecco L and Stecco C (2009) Fascial manipulation: Practical part. Padua: Piccin.

Stecco L and Stecco C (2013) Fascial manipulation for internal dysfunctions. Padua: Piccin.

Tesarz J, Hoheisel U, Wiedenhöfer B and Mense S (2011) Sensory innervation of the thoracolumbar fascia in rats and humans. Neuroscience 194 302–8.

Treatment of thoracic outlet syndrome and repetitive strain injury in a professional musician

Tiina Lahtinen-Suopanki, Finland

EDITOR'S COMMENT

Musicians are exposed to grueling physical and psychological demands, as maintaining performance quality over the duration of a public performance requires extremely long hours of practice. Pain from overuse can be debilitating and can even lead to giving up performing. This case report details treatment of a 30-year-old professional pianist who had progressively stopped playing concerts and could no longer play the piano for more than 10 minutes. The author, a physiotherapist with 38 years of experience and who is specialized in manual therapy and exercise medicine, first explains how her own clinical reasoning has changed since integrating Fascial Manipulation®–Stecco® method into her work. Details of how an apparently chronic musculoskeletal problem with neurological signs can be addressed through the Fascial Manipulation for Internal Dysfunctions (FMID) approach are then provided. Other aspects, such as the need to consider psychological stress, the interesting relationship between touch and memory, and the integration of different interpretations of the same dysfunction into one's practice, are also discussed.

Author's background

My physiotherapy clinical practice started in 1979, and my main interest has always been musculoskeletal physiotherapy. Having specialized in orthopedic manual therapy (OMT) in Norway (1987), I completed a bachelor's degree in health sciences at the University of Eastern Finland in 2014, with exercise medicine as the main subject. I currently work in a physiotherapy outpatient clinic where my clinical work is manifold: I do a lot of consulting for colleagues, medical doctors and other hospitals/institutions concerning chronic long-standing pain cases and unresolved cases,

and my caseload includes children, chronic pain patients, and professional athletes. I have also been a teacher of physiotherapists' ongoing education in manual and exercise therapy for over 30 years.

My motivation to understand the underlying factors behind dysfunctions that manifest as movement control disorders and non-specific pain has been the driving force behind continuing to seek out different explanations and treatment possibilities from those already available.

Experience with Fascial Manipulation®–Stecco® method

What I like to call 'my way' to Fascial Manipulation®–Stecco® method (FM) started in Zugliano, Italy, on the June 6, 2011, at 9 a.m., listening to Carla Stecco's lecture on fascial anatomy and physiology. I still remember the feelings and thoughts that arose during that lecture. How could the functional properties of a tissue that connects everything in the body have remained hidden for so long and, consequently, excluded from the practice of physiotherapy? As I listened the underlying factors behind 'non-specific' pain and the causes of movement control dysfunctions started to become clearer. Luigi Stecco's biomechanical model, which connects the motor unit, the joint, muscles, nerves, vascular components and fascia, was so logical that it made sense to start viewing human movement as the sum of all the active parts in synchrony. As a physiotherapist, I have always verified changes in motion, timing and possible tensional compensations. However, I usually started from the existing status, noticed the changes, and began to work on the problematic area. The ideas behind the FM model explained the need to find the reason for any given dysfunction. The whole procedure of collecting data, and especially the clinical reasoning behind a dysfunction, was elevated to another level from what I was previously used to in assessment. Throughout my working career, I have always sought out new explanations for dysfunctions, and manual therapy, therapeutic exercises, kinetic control, neurodynamics, Explain Pain concepts

(Butler & Moseley 2003) and so forth have all widened my spectrum of clinical reasoning. Of course, the patient's history and previous traumas have always been important but, after adding in the FM method of assessing a case, I have now understood what I call the 'big picture.' Why people with similar symptoms have such different reasons for their dysfunctions or people with similar traumas recover so differently has become clearer. I feel I have added a new perspective to my clinical reasoning.

Having practiced acupuncture since 1997, the myofascial unit viewpoint used in the FM approach was relatively easy to understand because the center of coordination (CC) points were already familiar. The connection from one point to the rest of the body, along with the diverse symptoms that patients describe, arising from somatic and autonomic nervous system dysfunctions that previously had been quite separate from each other, now had an anatomical explanation. Understanding the innervation of the fascia and its nervous connections to the central nervous system (CNS) provided logical explanations for the variety of difficult, long-standing, chronic situations I found daily in my patients. Fascial structures are densely innervated and, therefore, they provide a lot of input to the CNS. These structures can be a part of peripheral sensitization and, with prolonged bombarding of the CNS, they can also play a part in chronic pain states. Fascia surrounds all nerve structures, from the most peripheral areas to the spinal cord and vice versa. This makes it so interesting to trace the tensions underlying, for example, a 'thoracic outlet syndrome' or even numbness in a little finger. Adding knowledge of fascial anatomy and physiology to classical human anatomy and physiology studies, together with Stecco's biomechanical model, gives a totally new interpretation to many 'neurogenic' pain states. The results that I have had with chronic pain patients after adding the FM approach to my physiotherapy practice are far beyond what they were before. The only difficulty is to convince other medical personnel about the simple fact that fascia can play such an important role!

Motor control and neuromuscular training is an important part of physiotherapy intervention. Usually, movement control disorders are recognized and named and exercises are given to correct and normalize the situation. Having extensive experience as a physiotherapist for many professional athletes and dancers, I had often asked the question: Why does this person, who is really practicing and taking care of their musculoskeletal system, have a dysfunction that keeps coming back despite all the exercises and methods that are being applied? Furthermore, when even the most fine-tuned exercises were not bringing results it raised the question: What is lacking? The biomechanical model used in FM has been very helpful in understanding the connection between fascia, intramuscular and extramuscular receptors, and proprioceptors. It provides plausible explanations for inhibition and movement pattern changes, as well as for remote effects that different segments have on each other via the connecting fascial structures.

From a biopsychological viewpoint, it has been quite interesting to note how memories of long-forgotten traumas and accidents, fears and previous pain experiences can emerge during treatment of CCs and centers of fusion (CF). Post-traumatic dysfunctions often present as apparent musculoskeletal pain. The connection between the traumatized body part and the emotions evoked when that part is touched surprises the patient, and it very often represents the first step to recovery. This close relationship between fascial-orientated work and evoked emotions has also been a major step forward for me in the treatment of patients with long-standing pain states, particularly in those that have very sparse medical findings.

To summarize the main things that have changed in my physiotherapy practice since introducing the FM approach, I can say that both getting the 'big picture' in clinical reasoning and connecting the entire musculoskeletal system with the nervous system has moved my ability to help patients to a higher level. For these reasons, I have also trained to become an FM instructor, successfully completing my training in 2014. My teacher training has forced me study and to learn the FM approach thoroughly, essentially motivated by the idea of teaching others this highly effective method for helping people with dysfunction and pain.

Treatment of thoracic outlet syndrome and repetitive strain injury in a professional musician

Tiina Lahtinen-Suopanki

Thoracic outlet syndrome and repetitive strain injury in a professional musician

Introduction

E. is a 30-year-old pianist and piano teacher who has been playing the piano since she was 7 years old. The main hindrance to playing the piano is bilateral upper extremity pain, rapid fatigue, numbness varying between the second and fifth fingers, and lack of force in the fingers. Disability connected to playing the piano is 9 on the VAS scale and 4 for pain, burning, and tiredness.

Playing piano for 5–10 minutes and elevated arm positions provoke her symptoms. E. also feels that her left-hand fingers are clumsy when trying to perform rapid movements. These symptoms started 10 years ago after a period of intense training for a piano competition. She received physiotherapy and was asymptomatic for 2 years but the symptoms reappeared after another intense training period and, depending on the amount of playing, have been continuous for the last 5 years. She has not been able to continue her piano studies for the last 2 years. She has been diagnosed with thoracic outlet syndrome (TOS).

Concomitant pain

Concomitant dysfunctions include general joint laxity especially in the left shoulder (humerus: hu). E. feels that the whole left side of her body is 'tighter.' She wears an occlusion splint for nocturnal bruxism and occasionally has tenderness over her masticatory muscles bilaterally (caput: cp 2-3). She feels tightness in her thorax (th an), especially on the anterior of her sternum. Breathing feels heavy and she has voice problems, fatigue and tightness in the throat, mostly in the morning (cl). She also has sleep disturbances because of the pain. E. has had occasional low back pain (lumbar: lu), starting after a motor vehicle accident that occurred 6 years ago. She also suffers from dysmenorrhea (pelvis: pv), and she has lateral knee pain referring down both legs (ge-ta la bi) that is aggravated by walking.

Traumas, fractures and operations

E. was hit by a car 6 years ago and fell on her right side, hitting her head, which required sutures to her right forehead; she also had widespread bruising. She has had bilateral ankle sprains in her teen years, but there were no fractures or operations in her history.

Imaging studies

E. has had electromyography (EMG) twice in her upper extremities: 7 years previously findings were normal; 1 year prior to FM treatment there was mild conduction slowness of the ulnar nerve in the left cubital area.

Magnetic resonance imaging showed mild degeneration at the C4–5 and C5–6 levels.

One year ago, a Botox injection into the right anterior scalene muscle, performed by a hand surgeon as a preliminary trial for scalenotomy, proved to be ineffective.

Hypothesis

E. was referred for FM treatment because other rehabilitation interventions, including manual therapy (for neck and upper limbs), exercises (Pilates-type floor exercises), imagery training (pain, lateralization), sensory training (tubigrip, kinesiotape), graded exposure (timing of piano playing), and benign positional vertigo training (for tension) had all provided only short term or no symptom relief. FM was her last attempt at conservative treatment before having a right-sided scalenotomy.

I hypothesized that, with such extended and long-lasting symptoms in a highly motivated person, there had to be predisposing and maintaining factors other than just the local neck/arm area or the central sensitization, both of which had been focused on during previous interventions.

In FM, the person's entire data, present and previous, provide the baseline from which therapy is constructed.

First, I explained the FM procedure and, of course, peripheral and central pain sensitization mechanisms, and how everything that is going on in her system influences the 'big picture.'

My objectives in applying FM were to reduce the overall stress on the musculoskeletal system and the CNS and to create an environment for recovery.

Methodology

Movement verification (MoVe)

Movement verification (MoVe) was first carried out in the thorax, carpus, and talus segments (th, ca, ta). I chose these segments according to the presenting and concomitant pain areas, and the history. I could just as well have chosen the collum, pelvis, and digiti (cl, pv, di), but because a number of her symptoms could also point to internal fascial dysfunctions the th, ca, and ta segments were preferable, because the thorax is part of the abdominal canister and the ca and ta segments represent distal segments that can often be symptomatic with chronic internal dysfunctions. In addition:

- there was previous ankle trauma (ta) as well as referring pain from the lumbar segment to the talus (lu-ta)

- the carpus is a mobile segment between the elbow (cu) and finger (di) segments

- there were a lot of symptoms in the th segment and bilateral upper extremity symptoms can also be referred from there.

MoVe highlighted pain and movement limitations on the horizontal and frontal-plane, including weakness in the wrist or carpus (ca) movements in all the tested planes, plus pain and laxity/lack of muscle synchrony on the horizontal plane. There was very limited range of external rotation in the thorax (th) and it provoked her breathing problems bilaterally and tightness in the right supraclavicular area. All talus movements were asymptomatic and I added some other tests for the lumbar and pelvic segments that proved to be limited and painful.

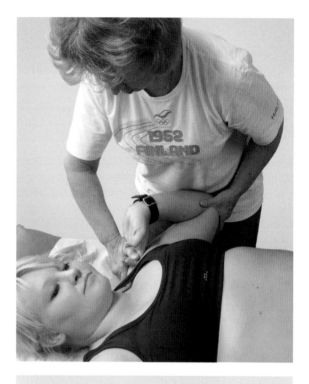

Figure 8.1
Neurodynamic test for the mechanosensitivity of the ulnar nerve on the left side

Neurodynamic tests were also performed and highlighted mechanosensitivity of the ulnar nerve and lower part of the brachial plexus during testing on the left side (Figure 8.1), and on both sides during the upper limb tension test 1 (ULTT 1).

Palpation verification (PaVe)

Palpation verification (PaVe) began with the thoracic segment. Due to prolonged pain and sensitization, E. was quite sensitive to all palpation and many non-densified points referred widely. The majority of densified points that caused referred pain similar to her symptoms were on the center of fusion points (CF). One thoracic center of coordination (CC) was also densified (er-th rt) and it referred a deep pain into the thorax area, triggering a memory of her breathing difficulties.

Treatment of thoracic outlet syndrome and repetitive strain injury in a professional musician

Tiina Lahtinen-Suopanki

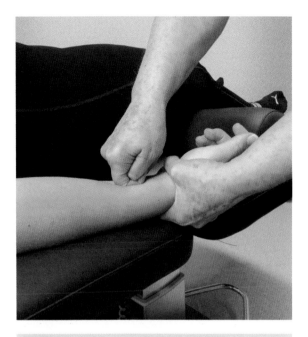

Figure 8.2
Palpation verification of the ante-latero-carpus center of fusion on the right side. This center of fusion is located on the flexor retinaculum on proximal part of distal third of the forearm, in the radial groove

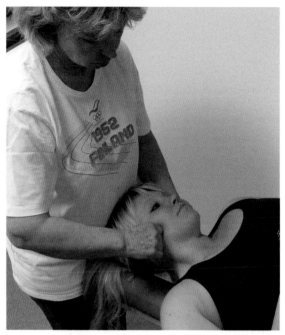

Figure 8.3
Manipulation of the ante-latero-caput 2 center of fusion on the right side. This center of fusion is located below the zygomatic arch, over the fascia of the masseter muscle

Palpation proceeded in the carpus segment (ca), where one CF on the right (an-la-ca1 rt) (Figure 8.2) was densified with deep pain and referral up to halfway on the forearm and back to the ulnar side of the palm. Plus, two CCs (la-ca rt and er-ca rt) were both densified, with strong referral to the dorsum of the hand, provoking feelings of numbness and weakness. Left me-ca was densified and provoked a feeling of cramps in her fourth and fifth fingers.

Treatment

Given the tenderness of numerous CFs and the widespread symptoms, in order to relieve tension throughout the whole system from the beginning, treatment was started according to the Fascial Manipulation for Internal Dysfunctions (FMID) guidelines.

1st treatment

The latero-lateral (LL) catenary was the most affected in the trunk, neck, and face, therefore, treatment started from this catenary. The LL catenary includes antero-lateral (an-la) and retro-lateral (re-la) CFs, as well as CCs from the lateromotion sequence. Treatment of a CC or CF continued until referred symptoms abated completely. Figures 8.3, 8.4, 8.5 illustrate a few examples of treatment positions. The location of some of the points that were treated and the symptoms that were provoked during treatment are also reported (Table 8.1).

2nd treatment

After 1 week, E. returned for treatment. She had been able to play piano for 40 minutes without symptoms and her breathing was easier and, therefore, treatment

CHAPTER 8

of the latero-lateral catenary was continued (Table 8.2). Further information about her history emerged little by little as treatment progressed, adding memories of previous symptoms and traumas.

3rd treatment

When E. returned for treatment after 2 weeks, she reported that she had been very tired and felt chills for 2 days

after the second treatment. However, she could now play forte and octaves for over 28 minutes, total playing time had increased to 50 minutes, and she had started to enjoy playing the piano again. She had also been jogging without pain in her knees. Therefore, I chose to treat the horizontal plane (ir and er) together with the antero-posterior catenary (AP), which includes antero-medial (an-me) and retro-medial (re-me) CFs (Table 8.3).

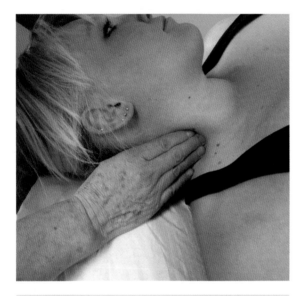

Figure 8.4
Location of the ante-latero-scapula 1 center of fusion on the right side, on the cervical fascia at the level of scalenus medius muscle

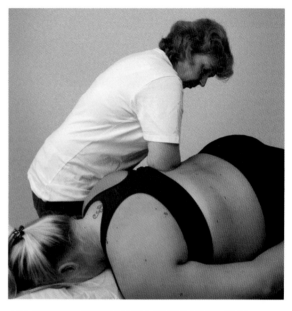

Figure 8.5
Manipulation of the retro-latero-lumbi center of fusion on the right side. This center of fusion is located on the thoracolumbar fascia (TLF) at the level of the 11th rib over the lateral raphe, at the attachment site of the latissimus dorsi muscle to the TLF

Table 8.1 1st Treatment

Points treated	Symptoms provoked
an-la-cp 2 rt	Right shoulder and throat pain
an-la-cl rt	Throat, right ear
an-la-sc1 rt	Ear, throat, feeling of fatigue in right upper limb
an-la-ta lt	Left shin and knee
re-la-th rt	All symptoms in right upper limb
re-la-lu lt	Increased tension and deep pain in pelvis
la-ca rt	Deep feeling in the carpus and palm
an-la-ca rt	Just tightness

Table 8.2 2nd Treatment

Points treated	Symptoms provoked
la-cl lt	
la-sc rt	
la-lu rt	
re-la-lu rt	Memory of a childhood trauma triggered quite a strong emotional reaction
an-la-pv 2 lt	Deep pain in the pelvis, similar to menstrual pain

Treatment of thoracic outlet syndrome and repetitive strain injury in a professional musician

Tiina Lahtinen-Suopanki

Table 8.3 3rd Treatment				
Points treated	re-me-th 1 and 3 lt	an-me-th 1 rt	an-me-cp 1 rt,	an-me-cp 2 lt
	ir-cp 3 rt	er-th rt	ir-pv lt	ir-sc rt

4th treatment

After another 2 weeks, I was able to treat the extremities, including the head/masticatory area and the hands.

Results

FM was applied for a total of seven sessions. In addition, I taught her relaxation techniques to cope with stress (bruxism), as well as exercises for the whole body to support her work as a musician.

Disability, pain, and fast fatigue related to piano playing decreased from VAS 9 to VAS 2–3, hand pain to VAS 1–2. The scalenotomy operation was cancelled. Range of motion (ROM) in the thorax was normal in all the directions. The difference in thoracic expansion between inhale and exhale (i.e., measurement of chest expansion motion on the T5 level) increased from baseline 3.5 cm to 5 cm, also allowing full and easy ROM for upper extremity movements. She was able to walk without knee pain and was able to jog for 30 minutes.

E. was able to continue her studies in piano playing and has already given concerts. She has occasional minor symptoms connected with prolonged playing but she manages them on her own by means of exercise and relaxation techniques and she is not scared of them anymore.

Discussion

During their career, which usually begins at a very early age, musicians' upper extremities are subjected to a vast number of repetitions and high load on the performing hands. This repetitive movement overloading can result in various symptoms, including deficits in motor control, loss of strength and endurance, numbness, tingling, and pain. The incidence of overuse syndrome among musicians is as high as 80% and even a minor clumsiness or numbness in a finger can end their career (Steinmetz et al. 2012).

The studies that have been done so far to identify the peripheral tissues and mechanics most involved in the production of such symptoms have focused on muscles, tendons, nerves, and the minor injuries and inflammation processes produced by the accumulation of repetitive stress (Barbe & Barr 2006; Fedorczyk et al. 2010). These studies have not included fascia in the pain-producing structures, even though it is a tissue that is present throughout the body, densely innervated with intrafascial free nerve endings and encapsulated receptors and autonomic fibers (Stecco C. et al. 2007; Stecco C. 2015) and it is involved in intra- and inter muscular force transmission (Huijing 2009; Yucesoy et al. 2010). Furthermore, it has been shown to be more sensitive to pain after exercise than muscle tissue (Lau 2015) and it is likely that fascia participates in proprioception and motor control (Stecco C. et al. 2011).

Mechanosensitivity and pain during playing is a common complaint, but clumsiness, lack of force, numbness, and tingling are just as common. At present the peripheral explanation for those complaints is not fully understood. In the absence of severe nerve compression (e.g., EMG findings) or other typical explanations for those symptoms, the situation can be very frustrating and fear-provoking for the person.

Musicians are often exposed to stressful situations in terms of long hours of practice, performing both before the public and under the constant scrutiny of conductors and, not the least stressful aspect, they are expected to perform perfectly every time. For example, while performing, bruxism is a typical symptom connected with stress. The constant overload of the masticatory muscles due to bruxism is common in musicians and it is associated with pain in the neck, shoulder, and hands (Steinmetz et al. 2012).

Over 30% of muscle contraction force is transmitted via the intramuscular and extramuscular fascial structures and every single note that the musician plays literally reverberates in these structures. The fascia is in direct continuity with Golgi tendon organs, the intrafusal and extrafusal fibers of muscle spindles, as well as mechanoreceptors embedded within the fascial tissues. Therefore, during playing, there is constant afferent information from the fascia to the CNS. Studies have shown that changes take place in fascial biomechanics due to overuse, traumas, and so forth, and these changes can influence motor control, produce a feeling of stiffness, lack of force and increased mechano-sensitivity during normal movements (Pavan et al. 2014; Stecco A. et al. 2016).

In E.'s case, neurodynamic tests highlighted mechanosensitivity of the ulnar nerve and lower part of the brachial plexus during testing on the left side, and on both sides during the upper limb tension test 1 (ULTT 1), which places tension mostly on brachial plexus. Neurodynamic tests tension the whole neurovascular canal, which includes the connective tissue or fascial components. The ulnar nerve passes through the medial intermuscular septum, which is tensioned by the contraction of muscle fibers that insert directly onto this septum. The septum is tensioned distally by flexor carpi ulnaris and pronator teres and proximally it is in direct continuity with the axillary/clavipectoral and supraclavicular fascia (Stecco C. 2015). Palpating points over the brachial plexus did provoke bilateral referred pain but this referral was not along specific nerve tracts. Instead, the pain was diffuse, and E.'s symptoms could be reproduced most precisely by palpating different CCs and CFs in the scapula and thoracic segments (in particular: la-sc bi, an-la-sc rt, re-la-th rt), meaning that referral to the upper extremities was not due to nerve compression on the nerve trunks as they pass between the scalene muscles or in the subclavian area, as is typically suggested with a diagnosis of TOS. It was hypothesized that the referred pain was due to the dysfunction and sensitivity of the fascial system as a result of prolonged tension in the head/cervical area (chronic bruxism) and repetitive stress of the upper extremities, together with fascial dysfunction in the trunk due to a previous trauma.

Conclusion

In this particular case, the patient perceived that the disability connected with her piano playing was a consequence of pain and rapid muscle fatigue. However, her recovery could be explained in terms of normalizing fascial biomechanics, which reconstitutes the afferent signals from intrafascial, muscle and tendon afferents, resulting in coordinated, smooth, pain-free movements.

Treatment of thoracic outlet syndrome and repetitive strain injury in a professional musician

Tiina Lahtinen-Suopanki

References

Barbe MF and Barr AE (2006) Inflammation and the pathophysiology of work-related musculoskeletal disorders. Brain, Behavior, and Immunity 20 (5) 423–9.

Butler D and Moseley L (2003) Explain pain. Adelaide: Noigroup Publications.

Fedorczyk JM, Barr AE, Rani S, Gao HG, Amin M, Amin S, Litvin J and Barbe MF (2010) Exposure-dependent increases in IL-1beta, substance P, CTGF, and tendinosis in flexor digitorum tendons with upper extremity repetitive strain injury. Journal of Orthopaedic Research 28 (3) 298–307.

Huijing PA (2009) Epimuscular myofascial force transmission: A historical review and implications for new research. Journal of Biomechanics 42 (1) 9–21.

Lau WY, Blazevich AJ, Newton MJ, Wu SS and Nosaka K (2015) Changes in electrical pain threshold of fascia and muscle after initial and secondary bouts of elbow flexor eccentric exercise. European Journal of Applied Physiology 115 (5) 959–68. doi: 10.1007/s00421-014-3077-5.

Pavan PG, Stecco A, Stern R and Stecco C (2014) Painful connections: Densification versus fibrosis of fascia. Current Pain and Headache Reports 18 (8) 441.

Stecco A, Stern R, Fantoni I, De Caro R and Stecco C (2016) Fascial disorders: Implications for treatment. PM & R 8 (2) 161–8.

Stecco C (2015) Functional atlas of the human fascial system. China: Churchill Livingstone, pp 234–72.

Stecco C, Gagey O, Belloni A, Pozzuoli A, Porzionato A, Macchi V, Aldegheri R, De Caro R and Delmas V (2007) Anatomy of the deep fascia of the upper limb. Second part: Study of innervation. Morphologie 91 (292) 38–43.

Stecco C, Stern R, Porzionato A, Macchi V, Masiero S, Stecco A and De Caro R (2011) Hyaluronan within fascia in the etiology of myofascial pain. Surgical and Radiologic Anatomy 33 (10) 891–6.

Steinmetz A, Möller H, Seidel W and Rigotti T (2012) Playing-related musculoskeletal disorders in music students-associated musculoskeletal signs. European Journal of Physical and Rehabilitation Medicine 48 (4) 625–33.

Yucesoy CA, Baan G and Huijing PA (2010) Epimuscular myofascial force transmission occurs in the rat between the deep flexor muscles and their antagonistic muscles. Journal of Electromyography and Kinesiology 20 (1) 118–26.

Fascial Manipulation® for Internal Dysfunction (FMID) in the treatment of chronic polyuria

Jaroslaw Ciechomski, Poland

EDITOR'S COMMENT

In classical medicine, it is rare to combine all the different symptoms of a patient into a single, logical, and causal sequence that leads to the formation of a disorder. In this chapter, the author, who is both a physiotherapist and an osteopath, initially explores the basic principles of osteopathy and outlines how the Fascial Manipulation®–Stecco® method, in particular the internal dysfunctions (FMID) approach, can be applied within the context of osteopathic philosophy. He then presents a case report concerning chronic polyuria in a 29-year-old woman. This is an interesting example of how a dysfunctional fascial system can apparently affect the functions of many organs in our body and how a dysfunction can be hypothesized on the basis of the patient's history, including events that may have occurred many years prior to examination. Furthermore, knowledge of the relationship between the fascial system and the autonomic nervous system can help to explain a multitude of clinical symptoms that patients present. This author has been fundamental for the introduction and spread of the FM method in Poland.

Author's background

After graduating as a physiotherapist from the Poznan University (Poland) in 1995, I worked as a researcher at the department of physiotherapy and physical medicine of this same university from 1996 to 2007, completing my doctorate in physiotherapy in 2003. I qualified as an osteopath in 2009 and subsequently became a Doctor of Osteopathic Medicine (DO) in 2011. Since 2000 I have taught 'Soft tissue therapy,' a postgraduate course accredited by the Polish Society of Physiotherapy. I first started studying Fascial Manipulation®–Stecco® (FM) method in 2007 and qualified as a teacher in 2012. Jostling between a busy private practice and a lively family life, in my spare time (*sic*), I am editor-in-chief of the *Practical Physiotherapy and Rehabilitation* journal.

Introduction

While the classical allopathic approach usually concentrates on symptomatic treatment, such as antibiotics for an infection, painkillers for pain, and strengthening exercises for muscle weakness, this type of approach makes it very difficult to understand all the interactions that occur within each person. In clinical practice, osteopaths often encounter many concurrent problems in the same patient and a holistic view is crucial to solving these problems.

Luigi Stecco's biomechanical model for the human fascial system is one of the few concepts that approaches treatment holistically. Having practiced osteopathy for many years and FM for more than 10 years, I have found the latter to be very effective for treating many disorders, including internal organ dysfunctions. Its precise analysis of fascial system functions combined with an interpretation of symptoms is unique and extremely helpful in osteopathic treatments.

In this chapter I hope to highlight the similar goals of osteopathy and FM and the relationships between these systems, and to encourage readers to study the Stecco method more deeply. In order to discuss both systems in reference to a clinical case, I will first present the basics of osteopathy.

Basic principles of osteopathy

Osteopathy is not a two-dimensional mechanistic approach. Viewing the body as a complex 'Meccano set' is not what osteopaths are about! Osteopaths see the body as a place where mind, body, and spirit interact and are reciprocally related, and where the building blocks of the body (the tissues) interact with, influence, and are influenced by internal physiology and homeostasis.

The founder of the osteopathic profession, Andrew Taylor Still, MD, DO, recognized that the state of health is a continuum from perfect function to complete breakdown. One of Still's basic beliefs about function was that the body is a totally integrated unit, its structures working together harmoniously to produce a healthy state. Lacking that harmonious function, the body produces conditions that lead to loss of health, or disease. The various parts of the body are functionally interconnected, allowing for necessary adaptations when demands on the body change. This view requires that the supply and maintenance of organs, mainly the visceral structures, are functionally connected with the body's primary consumer of energy, the musculoskeletal system. This interrelationship has long been neglected in medical practice. The communicating systems of the body, including the immune, endocrine, and neural systems, provide these interconnections.

Function is necessarily compromised when a problem develops in the integrating systems of the body and the stage is set for a lowered state of health and, eventually, for disease to occur (Stone 2007).

Concept of total and primary osteopathic lesion

An osteopathic lesion is generally defined as being a restriction of the mobility of a structure. However, this definition is only relatively correct and requires refinement.

An osteopathic lesion is not so much judged by the amplitude of the movement, but by the *resistance of the tissues*. The characteristic sign of an osteopathic lesion is a *tissue barrier*. This includes such things as a blockage, a locking, or a distinct resistance of the structure when it is put under even small amounts of tension.

The elements that determine the mechanical barrier could include articular tightness, muscular contracture, fascial tension, intra-osseous rigidity, energetic cysts, or a creation of the mind.

The *scarring process of the connective tissue* is a histological process that clearly explains the physiological mechanism of all osteopathic lesions.

The reaction of scarring within ailing connective tissue creates an osteopathic lesion. This scarring process evolves systematically and includes three stages:

1. *Inflammation*. In contractile tissues, such as skeletal muscles, visceral and arterial smooth muscles and myocardium, this inflammatory stage is generally associated with muscle spasm. Edema and muscle spasm create excessive tension on the tissue, which constitutes the first stage of an osteopathic lesion.

   Regardless of its acute and, at times, dramatic characteristics, inflammation remains a physiological reaction that prepares for tissue repair. This is normally a reversible phase and reversal can be spontaneous or brought about with the help of either symptomatic treatment or, preferably, a more holistic approach.

2. *Fibrosis*. The fibrosis stage corresponds to the *tissue reorganization* that follows an important inflammatory stage that was either prolonged or recurrent. The collagen fibers of the affected connective tissue increase in number and will have a different orientation depending on the constraints of the tissue. This increase of collagen fibers creates an area of long-lasting, adhesive tissue.

3. *Sclerosis*. This is the final stage of a pathological scarring process, where tissue alterations and hardening increase due to reduced vascularization. Characterized by ligamentous or tendinous calcifications, exostoses, arterial sclerosis, and cutaneous keratosis, the sclerosis stage is not reversible (or very minimally reversible). However, osteopathic treatment generally improves the organism's capacity to adapt to this lesion by stabilizing and minimizing the initiated process of tissue degradation.

FMID in the treatment of chronic polyuria
Jaroslaw Ciechomski

The fixation process of a tissue lesion is not always such a linear process. The fibrosis stage may include aggravation of inflammation and different stages of the lesion may coexist within the same region.

To justify the necessity for a global osteopathic approach, we must note one fundamental, histological point: *connective tissue is the only cellular organization of the human body that has the ability to scar.*

This physiological characteristic of connective tissue implies that all anatomical structures of mesodermal origin may be prone to an osteopathic lesion. This includes structures such as bones, muscles, fasciae, and blood vessels. From this viewpoint, muscle contracture, fascial fibrosis, articular blockage, osseous bowing, dermal fixation, visceral adhesion, or arterial spasm are all different expressions of the same lesion process. This explains why it is so important to consider all connective tissue as potential sites for osteopathic lesions.

Etiology of the osteopathic lesion

Factors that can start the scarring process that leads to an osteopathic lesion include:

* physical traumas
* infectious pathologies: bacterial pathogens set off a defense mechanism, generating an inflammatory reaction
* stress: disturbing emotions, excessive worries, intellectual overload or any other kind of psychological distress can generate physical tensions in the body, which, if unresolved, can become osteopathic fixations.

The total osteopathic lesion

The total osteopathic lesion is the sum of all individual lesions that emerge during a general osteopathic examination and constitutes a complex physical pathological entity. Each individual lesion has a different interfering potential, and the sum of the individual lesions greatly affects the organism because all of the individual lesions are interrelated.

The primary lesion

The primary lesion is an individual osteopathic lesion that, in comparison with all the other lesions present during the examination of a given patient in a given moment, has the greatest degree of tissue resistance (Chauffour & Prat 2002).

In order to normalize a patient's numerous osteopathic lesions, it is not realistic to individually correct each one because the unnecessary duplication of adjustments would only have a disturbing effect on the body.

In osteopathy, the first or original lesion is the starting point for the chain of lesions. This is different for each person. The patient's history leads us to the symptoms (symptomatic lesion) and to the triggering event (original lesion).

The primary lesion is always the one found during the examination and it is determined, and effectively treated, in the 'here and now' of the examination. There is no reason to establish a treatment plan based on the diagnosis from the preceding visits. The total lesion must be considered as a unique space-time element. There will never be two treatments exactly the same.

Role of Fascial Manipulation® in osteopathic treatment

The FM motto 'Manus sapiens potens est' ('A knowledgeable hand is powerful'), means that the more a therapist's hand is supported by scientific knowledge, the more effective it will be, and this idea fits in perfectly with the osteopathic vision.

FM uses different manual approaches to stimulate fascial points, or small areas, based on the principle that fascia is the only pliable and malleable tissue in our body. Osteopathy also places importance on connective tissue scarring. Fascia interacts with muscle spindles within the musculoskeletal system, and it also interacts with the neuronal network of the internal organs, which indicates it is the tissue that truly connects all body parts. Healthy fascia is elastic, fluid and has a correct basal dimension. Each fascia forms according to the function that it conducts, fitting into the osteopathic maxim of the relationship between structure and function.

The anatomical studies generated from FM theory explain how muscular fascia in the limbs is structured according to the logic of the myofascial sequences, diagonals and spirals, while muscular fascia in the trunk also has a prime role as a container for internal organs. This second function is involuntary, involving interaction with tensioning of, or tension within the internal organs. Hence, densification of the fascia of the anterior trunk wall sometimes causes musculoskeletal dysfunction but, more frequently, it causes internal disorders.

Understanding the biomechanical model of FM helps to explain all the symptoms and interactions between the fascial system and body dysfunction.

For musculoskeletal disorders, FM considers the myofascial structures (myofascial (mf) sequences, diagonals, spirals), utilizing specific movement and palpation verifications to identify altered tissue requiring treatment. For internal dysfunctions, it considers organ-fascial units and the correlations between autonomic ganglia in the internal fasciae. As typical movement restrictions are often lacking with internal dysfunctions, therapists verify tissue changes along special lines of tension in the trunk and the extremities to decide where to work in order to release the fasciae connected to the symptoms.

By connecting the history of the patient and analyzing movement restrictions, therapists can choose the most important fascial structures to treat in each particular case. As in osteopathy, no two treatments are exactly alike.

The model used in FM has so many similarities with the osteopathic philosophy that it is a great tool to use in everyday osteopathic practice.

CASE REPORT

Fascial Manipulation® for Internal Dysfunctions in the treatment of chronic polyuria

Introduction

Musculoskeletal symptoms

J. K., a 29-year-old pharmacist, presented with a 2-year history of bilateral pain radiating from her neck to her hands, together with similar pain radiating from her pelvic region to her feet. She also complained about recurrent headaches in the frontal region, occurring three times a month over the last 15 years. All the symptoms were aggravated by stress and extended sitting or standing. Lumbar pain increased during the night.

Visceral symptoms

J. K. had a 2-year history of ongoing, uninterrupted bladder infection. Frequent urination every hour was actually her biggest torment. She was also under hormone treatment for endometriosis, which increased her headache and the numbness in her hands and feet.

Previous surgery: appendectomy in laparoscopy (1995).

Medical diagnosis

- Narrowed urethra
- Polyuria (frequent urination) with bladder detrusor-constrictor dysregulation
- Hypothyroidism
- Endometriosis
- Physical condition after appendectomy (1995).

Medications

J. K. was on medication for an overactive bladder (Omnic ocas (tamsulosin) 0.4 mg, Urorec (silodosin) 4 mg, Doxar (doxazosin) 4 mg, Betmiga (mirabegron) 50 mg, Ubretid (distigmine bromide) 5 mg, Vesicare (solifenacin succinate) 10 mg).

FMID in the treatment of chronic polyuria

Jaroslaw Ciechomski

Osteopathic diagnosis

Somatic system:

- pelvic dysfunction with pudendal nerve stimulation (S2–4)

- thoraco-lumbar, lower ribs dysfunction with splanchnic nerve stimulation

- thoraco-cervical, upper ribs dysfunction with stellate ganglion stimulation

- cervical dysfunction with phrenic nerve and occipitalis major stimulation

- cranial dysfunction with stimulation of the vagus nerve in the jugular foramen together with glossopharyngeal (IX), and accessory nerve (X). Fascial restriction around the vagus nerve

- secondary myofascial pain with trigger point activation.

Fascial Manipulation diagnosis

- viscerosomatic origin of the dysfunction

- urinary apparatus dysfunction

- endocrine apparatus dysfunction.

Hypothesis

It was hypothesized that stiffness of the visceral fasciae could have increased abdominal pressure in the peritoneum and influenced the pelvic floor and bladder muscles function, and that disruption of the delicate mechanisms that coordinate the flow of urine to the bladder was the main problem in this patient.

Methodology

Movement verification

Standardized FM tests did not highlight any movement restrictions; therefore, additional osteopathic tests were used to find the dysfunctional segment. These tests included:

- vertebral and rib motion tests (Figure 9.1) to identify most restricted segments

- compression test of the trunk and extremities compartments (Figure 9.2) to find the biggest increase of pressure in the fascial compartments.

The most restricted areas were compared in order to find the primary lesion, which was located in the pelvic region.

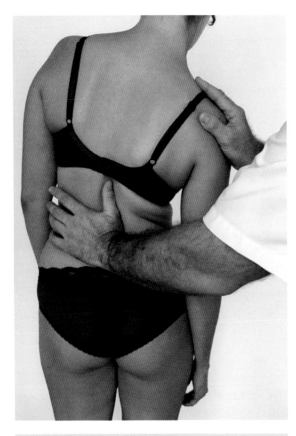

Figure 9.1
Vertebral motion test in standing. The test is useful to find the most restricted region

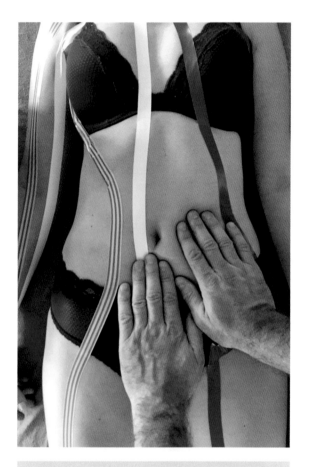

Figure 9.2
Pressure compression test. Example of the comparative analysis of the lower abdominal compartments (bladder and descending colon)

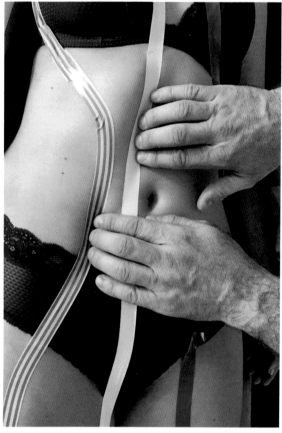

Figure 9.3
Palpatory verification of the trunk catenaries. The colored tapes indicate the pathway of the different catenaries (white: antero-posterior catenary, yellow-green: latero-lateral catenary, red: oblique catenary)

Palpation verification

The Fascial Manipulation® for Internal Dysfunctions (FMID) palpation verification procedure involved comparative palpation of principal centers of fusion (CFs) in the trunk (Figure 9.3) and of the control catenaries of the head. Palpation also included the pivot points (in the scapula and hip regions) and the distal tensor points (in the ankles and wrists).

FMID treatment

Three FMID treatments were performed over a period of 13 weeks. At each session, the CFs of the catenaries and pivot points, along with the distal tensor points in the ankles and wrists, were palpated.

FMID in the treatment of chronic polyuria

Jaroslaw Ciechomski

1st treatment: latero-lateral catenary (Table 9.1)

Table 9.1						
an-la-pv 1 rt	an-lu rt	an-la-th 2 lt,	an-la-cl rt	an-la cp 2 rt	an-la-sc 1 rt	an-la-ca 2 bi
an-la-ta 1 rt	an-la-cx rt	re-la-pv lt,	la-pv lt,	re-la-th lt	re-la-cp 3 bi	re-la-ta 2 lt

2nd treatment: oblique catenary (Table 9.2)

Table 9.2					
ir-pv rt	er-pv lt	ir-lu rt	ir-th rt	ir-cl rt	ir-cp 2 rt
ir-pe rt	ir-ca rt	er-pv lt	er-th rt	er-cx rt	er-ta lt

3rd treatment: anteroposterior catenary (Table 9.3)

Table 9.3				
an-me-pv 2 lt	an-me-th 2 lt, 1 bi	an-me-cl rt	an-me-cp 3 lt	an-me-sc 1 lt
me-sc lt	an-me-ca rt	an-me-ta 2 lt	an-me-cx rt	an-me-pe 3 rt

Results

After the first treatment, the patient reported a significant reduction in limb numbness and the urge to urinate. At the end of the three treatments, all the symptoms of tachycardia and numbness in the body were completely resolved. After almost 1 year, no symptoms had returned despite the fact that the patient had become pregnant during this time and had successfully given birth. Normally, pregnancy is one of the factors that increase urination, yet no deterioration in bladder function occurred. The patient was contacted several times by telephone in order to check her clinical condition and she has not needed any further treatment.

Discussion

Urination is a complex process involving different muscle groups and types, and an intricate nerve network located in the brain and spine, and in and around the bladder (Table 9.4).

Therefore, frequent urination can be a symptom of many different diseases and disorders, both physiological and psychological. The most common causes of frequent urination are diabetes, pregnancy, and prostate problems. Less common causes include anxiety, prostatitis, kidney infection, interstitial cystitis, overactive bladder syndrome and so forth.

Clearly, a differential diagnosis of frequent urination is essential to decide the appropriate treatment. Most importantly, unexplained and persistent frequent urination could be a symptom of something serious. For example, if the cause is diabetes, then treatment is focused on keeping blood sugar under control. If the cause is a kidney infection, then treatment usually comprises antibiotics and possibly painkillers.

Having excluded serious illness, polyuria is commonly diagnosed as 'overactive bladder syndrome', often associated with, as in this case, bladder detrusor-constrictor

Table 9.4 Summary of innervation of urination. Subject to voluntary facilitation and inhibition from higher brain centers				
Sympathetic innervation			**Parasympathetic innervation**	
Th12– L2	Activates sphincter, trigone and ureteral orifices Inhibits bladder wall		S2–4	Activates bladder wall Inhibits sphincter, trigone and ureteral orifices Peristalsis of distal part of ureters
Th10–11	Kidneys and ureters: vasoconstriction of afferent arterioles, decreases glomerular filtration rate, decreases urine volume		Fibers from vagus nerve	Kidneys Peristalsis of proximal part of ureters
			Pudendal nerve: somatic	
			Voluntary relaxation of external sphincter	

dysregulation. The origin of dysregulation has to be hypothesized from the patient's history.

In the case of J. K., it was hypothesized that the post-surgical status after appendectomy (performed 21 years previously) could have increased abdominal pressure in the peritoneum and influenced the pelvic floor and bladder muscle function.

Intra-abdominal pressure is normally 5–7 mmHg. Abdominal compartment syndrome (ACS), which can be iatrogenic from 10 to 12 mmHg, can provide an explanation for organ dysfunction. Many pathologies potentially cause an ACS, but that is not the subject here. However, some non-pathological but functional alterations can maintain a chronic substantial increase in abdominal pressure, exceeding the normal range and potentially leading to intra-abdominal hypertension.

During a laparoscopy, a pneumoperitoneum of 12–16 mmHg is achieved; therefore, abdominal pressure is increased. It has been demonstrated that abdominal pressure level can remain above the initial post-laparoscopy values (Jacobs et al. 2010). Other studies (Mazzocchi et al. 2010) show that pneumoperitoneum can cause damage to the integrity and biology of the peritoneum in animals and humans (Brokelman et al. 2011).

A number of experiments on animal models show that even a limited increase in abdominal pressure can cause bacterial translocation, in some cases independent of the type of gas injected during the pneumoperitoneum (Du et al. 2011). Additionally, cyclic compression produced in animals may alter the phenotype of vesical det-

rusor muscle cells, disrupting function (Gong et al. 2003). According to Schwarte (Schwarte et al. 2004), 'phenotypic transformation is the structural basis of functional changes of Detrusor Smooth Muscle cells subjected to periodic overload due to mechanical stretch.'

Furthermore, several authors (Hodges & Gandevia 2000; Hodges et al. 2007; Stecco L. & Stecco A. 2016) describe a specific postural alteration in chronic low back pain or sacroiliac pain concerning 'muscles in series': diaphragm-transversus abdominis-pelvic floor muscles. Represented both at peripheral and cortical levels, the action of these muscles should be integral, and they are simultaneously concerned with respiratory function and posture. These muscles in series can be chronically affected, even unilaterally, and they can present a number of anomalies such as delayed tensioning, fatigability, changes in cortical representation and so forth. These alterations cause a chronic disturbance in abdominal pressure, which remains slightly elevated when compared to a control group.

In J. K.'s case, releasing fascial tension by working on several catenaries (line of tension) could have decreased intra-abdominal pressure, resulting in improved bladder muscle function.

L. Stecco and C. Stecco (2014) describe the interrelationship between fasciae and internal organs in depth. Fasciae coordinate the micturition reflex: when the volume of urine exceeds approximately 300 ml, the perivesical fascia is stretched, which, in turn, stimulates the intramural neuronal network. Stretch of the bladder wall stimulates the sensory afferent fibers that transmit information to the spinal cord and the cerebral cortex.

FMID in the treatment of chronic polyuria

Jaroslaw Ciechomski

The central nervous system can either inhibit or permit the micturition reflex because it controls the external urethral sphincter via the pudendal nerve.

How parasympathetic and sympathetic impulses either inhibit or facilitate voiding to coordinate this mechanism is still not clear and it is somewhat controversial (Testut 1987). We need to question how the pudendal plexus, which has a parasympathetic origin, can activate contraction of the bladder's detrusor muscle and simultaneously inhibit the sphincter muscle? Normally, nerves only transmit impulses that activate rather than inhibit; therefore, it is difficult to understand how the same plexus can activate some muscles and inhibit others.

To explain this mechanism, we need to consider myogenic regulation, which is similar to intestinal regulation. When sympathetic stimulation of the bladder wall causes urine to enter the urethra, it dilates the fascial wall and this activates the myenteric neuronal network. The intramural neurons cause the smooth muscle behind the urine to contract and, by reflex, the musculature in front of the liquid relaxes. This mechanism propels the urine forward and it is interrupted at the level of external sphincter by voluntary contraction of skeletal muscles, such as the levator ani and pubococcygeus muscles.

It was hypothesized that J. K.'s main problem was due to stiffness of the fasciae that coordinate the flow of urine to the bladder causing disruption of this delicate mechanism. The gracilis muscle connects the bladder and lower limb fasciae and can pull on the obturator membrane and bladder ligaments, which could explain the numbness and pain experienced in her lower limbs.

To explain J. K.'s headache, upper limb pain, and hypothyroidism, the fascial connections with the endocrine apparatus require consideration. The thyroid gland's parenchyma is formed by glandular epithelium immersed in a connective tissue network called the stroma (Stecco L. & Stecco C. 2014). Innervation of the thyroid is sympathetic, and it also receives small nerve branches from the superior and inferior laryngeal nerves. In effect, all endocrine glands are innervated by three autonomic nerves: the vagus, phrenic, and splanchnic nerves, which are coordinated by fasciae that originate from the septum transversum. Communication between glands takes place via hormones secreting into the blood, which is a slow mechanism, and via the autonomic nervous system, which is coordinated by the glandular fasciae. The latter is a fast mechanism, needed in dangerous situations.

Endocrine glands are found in the head (hypophysis, pineal), neck (thyroid, parathyroid), thorax (thymus), lumbar region (pancreas, adrenals) and pelvis (gonads). These glands are united by a single fascia that begins from the sphenoid and descends with the stylohyoid muscle down to the hyoid bone. Here it splits to surround the thyroid and parathyroids, and then descends over the thymus and pericardium. The central tendon of the diaphragm is in direct contact with the liver and the adrenal glands. The transversalis fascia parts from the coronary ligament of the liver to surround the ovaries and the testicles in the pelvis. This fascial continuity explains the necessity to palpate points in all of the head, neck and trunk. The transversalis fascia is also sensitive to traction coming from distal tensors, located in the extremities of the limbs. Therefore, in pathological states, it can potentially generate pain in the limbs and head (Stecco L. & Stecco A. 2016).

Conclusion

1. There are many significant similarities between the osteopathic model and the FM model.

2. Application of the FM method allows for the interpretation of many clinical signs that have not been previously connected. It brings fast and lasting clinical effects and can be successfully used in osteopathic treatments.

3. There is a need for further studies in a larger population using the Stecco approach to confirm effectiveness and efficacy in the treatment of visceral dysfunctions.

CHAPTER 9

References

Brokelman WJ, Lensevelt M, Borel Rinkes IH, Klinkenbijl JH and Reijnen MM (2011) Peritoneal changes due to laparoscopic surgery. Surgical Endoscopy 25 (1) 1–9.

Chauffour P and Prat E (2002) Mechanical link. Fundamental principles, theory, and practice following an osteopathic approach. Berkeley, CA: North Atlantic Books, pp 26–30.

Du J, Yu PW and Tang B (2011) Application of stereology to study the effects of pneumoperitoneum on peritoneum. Surgical Endoscopy 25 (2) 619–27.

Gong Y, Song B, Jin Xy and Xiong EQ (2003) The relationship between phenotype transformation and biomechanical properties of detrusor smooth muscle cell subjected to the cyclic mechanical stretch. Zhonghua Wai Ke Za Zhi 41 (12) 901-5.

Hodges PW and Gandevia SC (2000) Changes in intra-abdominal pressure during a repetitive postural task. Journal of Physiology 522 (1) 165–75.

Hodges PW, Sapsford R and Pengel LH (2007) Postural and respiratory function of the pelvic floor muscles. Neurology and Urodynamics 26 (3) 362–71.

Jacobs JV, Henry SM and Nagle KJ (2010) Low back pain associates with altered activity of the cerebral cortex prior to arm movements that require postural adjustment. Clinical Neurophysiology 121 (3) 431–40.

Mazzocchi M, Dessy LA, Sorvillo V, Di Ronza S and Scuderi N (2010) A study of intraabdominal pressure modification in 'component separation' technique for repair of incisional hernia. Annali Italiani di Chirurgia 81 (6) 433–7.

Schwarte LA, Scheeren TW, Lorenz C, De Bruyne F and Fournell A (2004) Moderate increase in intraabdominal pressure attenuates gastric mucosal oxygen saturation in patients undergoing laparoscopy. Anesthesiology 100 (5) 1081–7.

Stecco L and Stecco A (2016) Fascial manipulation for internal dysfunctions: Practical part. Padua: Piccin, pp 154–5.

Stone CA (2007) Visceral and obstetric osteopathy. Edinburgh: Elsevier, Churchill Livingstone, ch 1, pp 4–5.

Testut L (1987) in Stecco L, Stecco A (2016) Fascial manipulation for internal dysfunctions: Practical part. Padua: Piccin, p 144.

Resolving partial nipple ischemic necrosis following nipple-sparing mastectomy

Natalie Brettler, Israel

EDITOR'S COMMENT

In this chapter, the author presents the resolution of a chronic post-surgical partial necrosis of the nipple area in a woman who had initially sought treatment for limited, painful shoulder and neck movements. A combination of manual techniques, which are all part of the Fascial Manipulation®– Stecco® approach, were used to treat the deep fascia and superficial fascia in this case. The deep fascia manual technique differs from that used in superficial fascia treatments and, even more specifically, manual techniques can vary between different superficial fascia dysfunctions. The results on the partial necrosis are well-documented photographically and anatomical details are also given concerning the points and the areas that were treated. While it is common for deep fascia work to reduce pain and free movement, the author suggests that the superficial fascia approach may have targeted skin vascularization more efficiently, improving blood flow and reducing necrosis dramatically.

Author's background

Having completed my degree in physiotherapy at the University of Haifa in Israel, I continued my studies with a range of postgraduate courses including Fascial Manipulation®–Stecco® method (FM), applied kinesiology, dry needling, treatment of vestibular disturbances, Pilates, Kinesio Taping® and so on. I initially worked in the public sector, mostly in the field of orthopedics. At present, I work in a private clinic in Tel Aviv specializing in orthopedics and sports rehabilitation. My patients range from non-professional sportsmen to Olympic level competitors, including Israel's national team of rhythmic gymnasts and with them I attended the Olympic Games in Rio de Janiero in 2016.

I qualified as an FM teacher in 2013, and I have been teaching courses, both in Israel and internationally (Russia, Slovakia, Philippines), conducting ongoing education workshops for colleagues, and presenting case reports at national and international conferences since then.

Experience with Fascial Manipulation®– Stecco® method

I was fortunate to come across the Stecco method in my early years as a physiotherapist. Most of what I learned at university and on the various postgraduate courses I had attended, regarding assessing and treating a patient, was focused locally at the patient's specific area of pain or dysfunction. I always felt like something was missing with this localized approach, which tries to associate a biomechanical abnormality with the patient's symptoms. What immediately inspired me in the Stecco method was the way in which it viewed the entire body as a functional and holistic unit, but with an anatomical and physiological explanation demonstrating the connection between the different segments/units of the body and how they integrate and work together. Another aspect that impressed me was the insistence of the Stecco approach to search for the source of the problem and not to only focus on the symptom.

As an analogy, when one has a leak somewhere in one's house, it is clear that the problem is from a fault in a pipe. It is obvious that one needs to wipe up the water on the floor but in order to fix the problem, the leak in the pipe needs to be closed up. Unfortunately, many methods of assessment and treatment do not aim to fix the leak in the pipe, but rather to wipe the floor clean, which at best will give temporary relief locally, but will not solve the real problem.

Another reason why I tend to prefer the FM approach is that there is no protocol to treatment. Every person that comes to the clinic, for example, with back pain, will receive a different treatment according to the compensatory patterns that their body has produced over time.

In all my years of work, I have never treated two people presenting with the same symptoms in the same manner. In order to find what the source of their problem is (the leak in the pipe) and what the body's compensation for this is (the water on the floor), each patient needs to be assessed individually according to their history. In this way, each individual patient receives the appropriate treatment. It sounds challenging to provide each patient with a unique treatment. The challenge is to solve the 'riddles' of the presenting symptoms and to figure out where the person's problem lies. In fact, the only thing that hurts an FM therapist at the end of the day … is their head!

Since I started working with this method, I feel that I see the body in three dimensions, not in two. My assessment and diagnosis is much more comprehensive and detailed than before, and therefore I find that my effectiveness in treatment is much more rapid and yields better results.

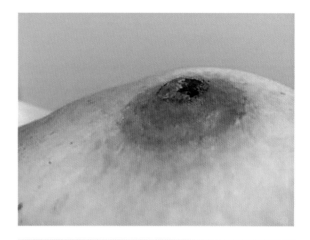

Figure 10.1
A lateral view of the patient's nipple before treatment

CASE REPORT

Resolving partial nipple ischemic necrosis complication by Fascial Manipulation®– Stecco® method following nipple-sparing mastectomy

Introduction

A 50-year-old woman was referred to my clinic specifically for a FM treatment due to pain in the right, posterior part of her shoulder, neck, and scapula. Her medical history included breast enhancement surgery using a silicone implant in 1996 without any complications. In 2014, she was diagnosed with right breast cancer and was treated by bilateral nipple-sparing mastectomy with immediate reconstruction.

On examination, partial ischemic necrosis of the right nipple was noted (Figure 10.1). On palpation, rigidity of the breast (right breast more than left) was felt, with the patient reporting a decrease in sensation of the breast area, including the nipple, as well as pain and a sense of

pulling on the breast area during shoulder flexion and external rotation. The nipple was flat and non-erectile and, due to the poor appearance of the right nipple, she had taken the surgeon's advice to have a tattoo around the nipple in order to make the nipple look more aesthetically pleasing (Figure 10.2). There was also a rough scar around the right nipple and the axilla where there had been a drain after the mastectomy surgery. It is important to note that this woman approached me in my role as a physical therapist, hoping I could help her to resolve her musculoskeletal pain, and not for a treatment of the necrosis of the nipple because she had been told that there was nothing that could be done for this complication.

I immediately accepted to treat this patient using the FM method as, due to the variety of symptoms she presented, it was deemed appropriate.

Breast cancer is the most common cancer in women in developed countries (Ginsburg et al. 2017). Thanks to a variety of new treatments, the survival rate of women with breast cancer has increased significantly (Siegel et al. 2016). However, due to the treatments, these women may develop a variety of complications such as decreased range of motion of the upper limb and neck, pain syndromes, muscle atrophy, and lymphedema

Resolving partial nipple ischemic necrosis following nipple-sparing mastectomy

Natalie Brettler

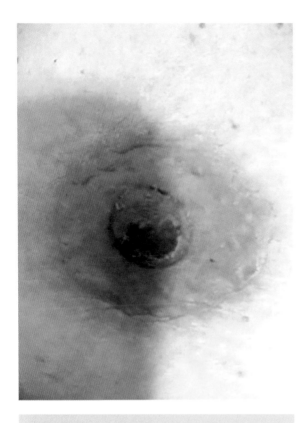

Figure 10.2
A frontal view of the patient's nipple before treatment

(DiSipio et al. 2013). As a result of these complications, they experience a decline in their quality of life, a reduction in their hours of work, and an inability to partake in sports and other recreational activities (Stecco L. & Stecco C. 2014; Stecco C. 2015).

Nipple-sparing mastectomy is a surgical technique that preserves the patient's nipples as well as the areolar skin. The removal of the breast tissue leaves an envelope of skin that can be filled with either an implant or tissue from another part of the patient's body. Preserving the nipple has significant benefits such as an improved aesthetic outcome and psychosocial well-being. However, these women can unfortunately suffer from postoperative complications, with incidence rates ranging from 3% to 37%, depending on which article one reads. The most

frequent complications are skin and/or nipple necrosis, partial or full loss of pigmentation of both nipple and areola, and the need for tattoos to provide artificial pigmentation and better appearance. Furthermore, reconstructed nipples are usually insensate and non-erectile.

Hypothesis

This patient presented complications in both her right arm and her shoulder, as well as the nipple. Treatment of this patient needed to focus on improving blood supply to the nipple and areola areas, as well as reducing pain and improving range of movement (ROM) in the shoulder. The thorax segment was hypothesized to be the likely source of the shoulder and neck pain, as well as being clearly involved in the other complications such as necrosis, loss of sensation, and lack of nipple erection. FM was considered to be suitable as a treatment method because it includes manual techniques that focus on both the deep and the superficial fascia, therefore it has the potential to address all the concomitant presenting components.

Methodology

After thoroughly examining the patient's history using the method specific FM assessment chart, I assessed the chest area, examined the sensation in both breasts and, due to the patient's complaint of shoulder and neck pain, performed movement tests for the humerus (HU) and collum (CL) segments. Flexion and horizontal adduction of the HU and left and right rotation of the CL segment were all painful and limited. After recording the findings (using both photography and writing), I began to palpate the centers of coordination (CC) and centers of fusion (CF). I chose two segments to palpate in order to find a line of tension. The two selected segments were the thorax (TH) and the humerus (HU). The TH was chosen also because it was the segment in which she underwent the mastectomy, as well as the reconstruction surgeries. The HU segment was chosen as this was the site of pain (SiPa), or the main area of pain that the patient complained about.

On comparative palpation of the chosen segments, the most involved plane was found to be the horizontal plane, and the ante-latero (an-la) and retro-medio (re-me) myofascial diagonals were also implicated. I then extended palpation to other segments, including CL, scapula (SC), and cubitus (CU), but only on the horizontal plane and the mf diagonal lines of an-la and re-me. It seemed that the CFs on the diagonals were more densified than the horizontal CCs. Therefore, the diagonals were chosen for the first treatment.

1st treatment

The points that were treated in this session combined myofascial diagonals on both sides of the body in order to balance the diagonal lines of tension (Table 10.1).

Result after 1st treatment

Immediately after the treatment the involved segments were retested and there was a significant decrease in the visual analog scale (VAS) pain score in movements of both segments. More specifically, pain on flexion and horizontal adduction of the HU decreased from 8 to 2. Pain in the CL with both left and right rotation decreased from 7 to 1. The sensation of pulling in the posterior part of the scapula also decreased. The next treatment was scheduled for the following week.

One week after the first session, there was a significant change in the appearance of the nipple area (Figure 10.3). The ischemic area disappeared, the rigidity of the breast decreased, and the patient reported that there was an increase in the sensation of the breast area. In addition, the pain experienced with shoulder flexion and external rotation had decreased by 70%.

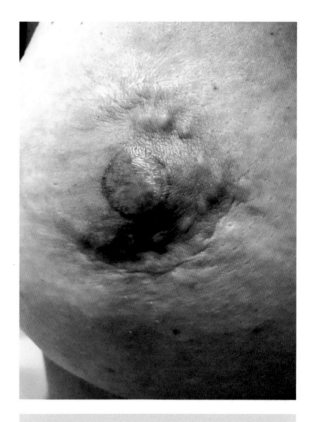

Figure 10.3
The nipple of the patient a week after the first treatment

After working on the deep fascia in the first session, both the superficial and deep fascia were treated in the second session because subcutaneous nerves, blood vessels, and the lymphatic system are all found in the superficial fascia.

The Fascial Manipulation for Internal Dysfunctions (FMID) approach addresses the superficial fascia more

Table 10.1 1st Treatment and anatomical location of treated points				
an-la th 1 bi	an-la cl rt	an-la hu rt	re-me th 2 bi	re-me sc rt
4th intercostal space, midway between mamillary and axillary lines	Posterior to angle of the mandible, over antero-lateral fibers of the sternoleidomastoid (SCM) muscle	Proximal 1/3 of the arm, on the antero-lateral fibers of deltoid, distal portion	Longitudinal paravertebral sulcus, from T4 to T6	Superior medial border of the scapula, over the tendon of rhomboid minor

specifically, utilizing appropriate manual techniques that can influence superficial blood flow (see Discussion). Based on the anatomical organization of the retinacula cutis (collagenous septa that extend between the skin and the superficial fascia and this fascial layer and the underlying deep fascia), the hypodermis, which includes the superficial fascia is divided into so-called 'quadrants' (Stecco L. & Stecco C. 2014). In effect, the retinacula cutis layers in the trunk and limbs present some longitudinal and horizontal reinforcements, which divides the superficial fascia into compartments or quadrants. It should be noted that, when recording superficial fascia treatment, each specific quadrant is indicated by the letter 'q' to distinguish it from a center of fusion.

2nd treatment

This treatment involved working the superficial fascia in several quadrants using a specific manual technique for this fascial layer, as well as treating some CCs on the horizontal plane, using the typical FM deep friction technique for the deep fascia (Table 10.2).

Results

A week after the second session, the color of the nipple became lighter and its shape was rounder (Figure 10.4). The patient reported a normal feeling in the breast and nipple area and that she had no pain during shoulder flexion and external rotation.

A follow-up with the patient 6 months after treatment, as well as 1-year post treatment, showed that the results of the treatment were long-lasting.

Discussion

Between 25% and 60% of surviving patients who have undergone surgery for breast cancer experience persistent postsurgical pain. In a prospective Australian study,

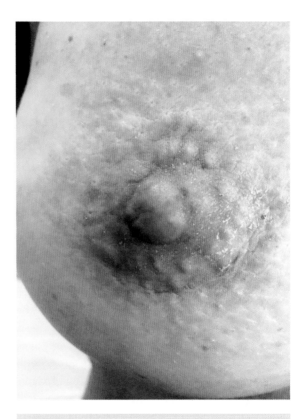

Figure 10.4
The nipple of the patient a week after the second treatment

Table 10.2 2nd Treatment, including anatomical location of relevant quadrants and CCs

q-an-me-sc rt	q-an-me-th rt	q-an-me-hu rt	ir th rt
From inferior margin of clavicle to the transverse nipple line	From inferior border of manubrium to superior margin of xiphoid process	From anterior border of acromion to the axillary cavity	5th and 6th intercostal spaces, on the mammillary line
ir sc rt	er th bi	er hu rt	
Inferior to middle 1/3 of clavicle, over subclavius and upper fibers of pectoralis major	Superior 1/3 of medial border of scapula at the level of scapular spine	Level of humeral head, over the posterior aspect of the deltoid	

62% of the population still suffered from at least one impairment as a complication of breast cancer treatment and 27% suffered from two to four impairments after 6 years (Wang et al. 2016). These complications can include persistent pain, skin and/or nipple necrosis, partial or full loss of pigmentation of the nipple, loss/decrease of sensitivity and erectness of the nipple, arm lymphedema, and shoulder and arm morbidities (restricted range of motion, pain, and arm volume changes) (DiSipio et al. 2013).

There is a limited description in literature of a suggested conservative treatment for these complications. Manual lymph drainage in combination with physical exercise is recommended for breast cancer patients in preventing post-mastectomy scar formation, upper limb lymphedema, and shoulder joint dysfunction (Zhang et al. 2016).

For postoperative nipple-areolar complex (NAC) necrosis, the literature suggests saline dressing or antibiotic topical cream. One article reported that using hyperbaric oxygen therapy had good results (Alperovich et al. 2015). All other treatments suggested for necrosis are surgical, with a long healing process and results that are not aesthetically pleasing.

The skin is sensitive to various types of external stimuli including tactile, pressure, thermal, and painful stimuli, all of which are perceived by specific cutaneous nerve endings. If the superficial fascia densifies, causing compression of afferent nerves, cutaneous sensitivity is distorted, giving rise to local numbness and anesthesia (Stecco L. & Stecco A. 2016), as in this patient's case. Furthermore, skin vascularization is strongly affected by the superficial fascia because of its anatomy (Stecco A. et al. 2016). All the subcutaneous arteries form two subcutaneous plexuses: the subpapillary plexus, just under the papillary dermis (top layer of the skin), and the deep plexus, which is inside the bilamellar superficial fascia layer. The arteries of the deep plexus have multiple arteriovenous connections, providing shunts that control blood flow to the skin and, consequently, body temperature. The

dilation and narrowing of the subcutaneous arteries determines both skin temperature and color.

It is possible that a change in the superficial fascia (such as densification or fibrosis) could restrict or constrict the arteries inside it, causing a change in skin color, reducing skin vascularization and even resulting in chronic ischemia of the skin (Distler et al. 2007; Stecco C. 2015).

During cancer surgery, the superficial fascia of the pectoral area and axilla are always damaged or removed (partially or totally) because of the intimate adherence between the superficial fascia and the inner side of the mammary gland, creating a scar in the subcutaneous tissue and damaging the sliding system between the different layers (superficial fascia, deep fascia, and muscles).

Between the superficial fascia and the deep fascia of the thorax there is loose connective tissue that normally permits the movement of the mammary gland with respect to the underlying muscular plane.

The deep fascia of the trunk is very different from that of the limbs. In the limbs, deep fascia is easily separable from the underlying muscles because, due to their epimysial fascia, the limb muscles are mostly free to slide under the deep fascia. In the trunk, there are three muscular planes that are covered with three fascial layers and are separated by loose connective tissue that permits the sliding between the different muscular layers. In particular, the fascia of the more superficial muscular layer is thinner and it adheres strongly to the muscle; the fascia in each layer is also layer-specific because it continues to cover all the muscles in the same layer. This particular anatomy in the trunk region allows peripheral motor coordination and proper transition of force to the upper and lower limbs.

After breast surgery, densification and/or fibrosis can occur in the trunk, altering the loose and dense connective tissue, affecting the sliding motion of the muscular and fascial layers one upon another and causing myofascial dysfunction. This myofascial dysfunction can be expressed in arm comorbidity due to the continuation of the fascia of the trunk with that of the limbs. The anatomy of the myofascial layers of the trunk could explain the pain that the patient in this case study had during shoulder movements, as well as the pulling sensation in her breast during arm movements.

Conclusion

Surgical treatment of breast cancer can cause a variety of complications such as: decreased range of motion of the upper limbs and neck, pain syndromes, muscle atrophy, lymphedema and necrosis. While all of the complications mentioned above, except necrosis, are usually treated with physical therapy and various manual therapies, there is no literature-documentation for treating necrosis with manual therapy. This chapter presents a documented treatment of manual therapy for partial necrosis using the FM method. The goal of this chapter is to present therapists and patients with the benefits of using this method for improving vascularization and to encourage further research in this field.

References

Alperovich M, Harmaty M and Chiu ES (2015) Treatment of nipple-sparing mastectomy necrosis using hyperbaric oxygen therapy. Plastic and Reconstructive Surgery 135 (6) 1071–2.

DiSipio T, Rye S, Newman B and Hayes S (2013) Incidence of unilateral arm lymphoedema after breast cancer: A systematic review and meta-analysis. The Lancet Oncology 14 (6) 500–15.

Distler JH, Jüngel A, Pileckyte M, Zwerina J, Michel BA, Gay RE, Kowal-Bielecka O, Matucci-Cerinic M, Schett G, Marti HH, Gay S and Distler O (2007) Hypoxia-induced increase in the production of extracellular matrix proteins in systemic sclerosis. Arthritis and Rheumatism 56 (12) 4203–15.

Ginsburg O, Bray F, Coleman MP, Vanderpuye V, Eniu A, Kotha SR, Sarker M, Huong TT, Allemani C, Dvaladze A and Gralow J (2017) The global burden of women's cancers: A grand challenge in global health. The Lancet 389 (10071) 847–60.

Siegel RL, Miller KD and Jema A (2016) Cancer statistics, 2016. CA A Cancer Journal for Clinicians 66 (1) 7–30.

Stecco A, Stern R, Fantoni I, De Caro R and Stecco C (2016) Fascial disorders: Implications for treatment. PM & R 8 (2) 161–8.

Stecco C (2015) Functional atlas of the human fascial system. Edinburgh: Churchill Livingstone, Elsevier.

Stecco L and Stecco C (2014) Fascial manipulation for internal dysfunctions: Theoretical part. Padua: Piccin.

Stecco L and Stecco A (2016) Fascial manipulation for internal dysfunctions: Practical part. Padua: Piccin.

Wang L, Guyatt G, Kennedy S, Romerosa B, Kwon H, Kaushal A, Chang Y, Craigie S, Almeida C, Couban R, Parascandalo S, Izhar Z, Reid S, Khan J, McGillion M and Busse J (2016) Predictors of persistent pain after breast cancer surgery: A systematic review and meta-analysis of observational studies. Canadian Medical Association Journal 188 (14) 352–61.

Zhang L, Fan A, Yan J, He Y, Zhang H, Zhong Q, Liu F, Luo Q, Zhang L, Tang H and Xin M (2016) Combining manual lymph drainage with physical exercise after modified radical mastectomy effectively prevents upper limb lymphedema. Lymphatic Research and Biology 14 (2) 104–8.

Treatment of Bell's palsy

Larry Steinbeck, USA

EDITOR'S COMMENT

This case study addresses treatment of Bell's palsy, a condition affecting the seventh cranial nerve, also known as the facial nerve, which results in an inability to control the facial muscles on the affected side. Treatment includes a combination of specific techniques for the deep fascia and the superficial fascia. Given that the superficial fascia of the face envelops and connects all the mimic muscles, creating an organized fibrous, muscular network, and that the deep fascia envelops the masticatory muscles, including the temporalis and masseter, as well as the salivary glands, both fascial layers merit attention following Bell's palsy. All of the muscles involved in chewing and swallowing are interconnected by fasciae, therefore, a normal tensional relationship in this fascial network is essential for correct function. The author, one of the participants in the first English course of Fascial Manipulation® held in Italy in 2010, discusses the possible implications of densification in these two tissues and how it may impede the restoration of nerve and muscular function.

Author's background

I graduated from Ball State University, in Muncie, Indiana, with a Bachelor of Science degree in physical therapy and a minor in athletic training in 1985. The following year, I earned a Master of Science degree in physical education from Ohio University with an emphasis on athletic training, while simultaneously achieving the high honor of becoming a licensed physical therapist and also a certified athletic trainer through the National Athletic Trainers Association.

Initially, my professional practice focused on the amateur athletic population along with post-surgical reha-

bilitation. As my career evolved I became interested in the treatment and care of the geriatric population, and the majority of my career has been devoted to treating the adult population with acute and long-standing pain. Certifications include dry needling techniques through Myopain Seminars® and Fascial Manipulation® (FM) through the Fascial Manipulation® Association. I am an approved instructor for the Level I and II courses for FM and I currently work full-time in an outpatient rehabilitation clinic that is located in Jasper, Georgia.

Experience with Fascial Manipulation®– Stecco® method

While attending Ohio University I had the opportunity to spend time at their College of Osteopathic Medicine and to observe the physicians who still integrated manual medicine into their practices. This experience introduced me to osteopathic manipulative techniques, including muscle energy techniques, thrust manipulation, myofascial release, strain/counterstrain, and craniosacral therapy. I gravitated toward myofascial release and strain/counterstrain and had the opportunity to pursue this further with Robert Ward (DO) at Michigan State University, as well as strain/counterstrain through Harold Schwartz (DO) in continuing education courses. Dr Ward used a term that I appreciated when he would refer to the 'neuromusculoskeletal biomechanical system.' I was intrigued by the interconnectivity of the muscular and fascial systems and continued to study their interrelationship. It was while attending a dry needling course through Myopain Seminars® that I stumbled across a reference to a scientific paper by Carla Stecco. I asked others in the course if they were familiar with this study regarding fascial histology and architecture. They were not aware of it, and this inspired a dialogue and further research/study on my part. I really appreciated how their numerous papers provided a fresh, more detailed view and interconnectivity of what I knew as the 'neuromusculoskeletal biomechanical system.' I had studied works from other authors that linked 'total body' connectivity, but none were as detailed and/or related to motor control and proprioception as the work of the Steccos. As I studied the model that Luigi Stecco had originated, I appreciated that it appeared seamless with regards to global assessment and treatment methodology. There were no unique rules based on a given body part or segment involved. It did not matter if you were evaluating the head and neck or the ankle and foot, the same principles were applied. There were no particular 'tricks' that needed to be deployed for a specific problem. It was quite consistent in logic and presentation. Through the fascial architecture description and its relationship with muscles I could comprehend and appreciate a better explanation for other methods/models that I was using. I had a greater understanding of why joint mobilization, thrust manipulations, or proprioceptive neuromuscular facilitation could be effective, as I realized that it is right there in the 'neuromyofascial skeletal biomechanical system.'

CASE REPORT

Fascial Manipulation®–Stecco® method for the treatment of Bell's palsy

Introduction

R. V., a 72-year-old male, presented with a diagnosis of Bell's palsy. He reported primary limitations of an inability to close the right eye and drooling while consuming beverages. He was only able to drink by using a straw and, as he has said, 'it was not the proper way to have a glass of wine!' There was no associated pain, but he did have irritation in his right eye from 'dryness' that was somewhat alleviated with the use of ointments. Symptoms had been present for almost 5 months prior to coming for treatment and he reported that there had not been any appreciable change in motor function since the Bell's palsy diagnosis was first made. He had completed three prescriptions of oral corticosteroids and one prescription of antivirals.

Bell's palsy can be a challenge to treat, as there is no consensus for the etiology of signs/symptoms, which range from herpes simplex virus to mononeuropathy akin to Guillain–Barré and due to nerve compression. According to the Canadian Medical Association's guidelines for treatment of Bell's palsy (de Almeida et al. 2014), there is strong confidence associated with the use of corticosteroids and antivirals (when they are used in conjunction with corticosteroids as opposed to antivirals alone) in severe cases. They note weak confidence when using electrical stimulation or surgical decompression in acute cases and offer no advice with regards to exercise therapy in acute cases.

This patient was referred for treatment by friends who had had successful resolution of other musculoskeletal diagnoses with FM treatments.

Hypothesis

Due to the length of time that symptoms had been present in this case without any significant change in motor function, it was hypothesized that there was no longer any active inflammation or virus delaying the return of the motor component of the facial nerve. FM was chosen because of its model on impacting proprioception through the muscular/fascial interface and indirectly impacting tension on local nerves. By altering the tension through the superficial musculoaponeurotic system (SMAS) in addition to the muscles associated with the head and neck, it was hypothesized that FM might be effective in restoring motor control and at the same time limiting potential synkinesis. Synkinesis is a common sequel to Bell's palsy and it is defined as an involuntary movement associated with a given expression. As an example, a person with Bell's palsy might experience a persistent inability to keep their eye open when smiling. Another example common among people who have Bell's palsy is the inability to disassociate eyelid opening/closing, in which eyelid movement only occurs bilaterally and not independently.

Methodology

Upon initial assessment, the House–Brackmann facial nerve grading scale was utilized as an outcome measure (Table 11.1). This case rated a grade V on this scale.

Treatment of Bell's palsy

Larry Steinbeck

Table 11.1 House–Brackmann grading system. Modified from Sun et al. (2002)					
Grade	Description	Characteristics			Estimated function (%)
		Gross	At rest	Motion	
I	Normal	Normal	Normal	Normal	100
II	Mild dysfunction	Slight weakness noticeable on close inspection, may have very slight dyskinesia	Normal symmetry and tone	Forehead: moderate to good, eye complete closure w/minimum effort; mouth slight asymmetry	80
III	Moderate dysfunction	Obvious but not disfiguring difference between two sides: noticeable but not severe synkinesis, contracture, and/or hemifacial spasm	Normal symmetry and tone	Forehead: slight to moderate movement; eye: complete closure w/effort; mouth: slightly weak w/maximum effort	60
IV	Moderately severe dysfunction	Obvious weakness and/or disfiguring asymmetry	Normal symmetry and tone	Forehead: none; eye: incomplete closure; mouth: asymmetric w/maximum effort	40
V	Severe dysfunction	Only barely perceptible motion	Asymmetry	Forehead: none; eye: incomplete closure; mouth: slight movement	20
VI	Total paralysis	Total paralysis	Asymmetry	No movement	0

Movement verification (MoVe)

The patient presented with gross, barely perceptible motion, right/left asymmetry at rest, no right forehead movement, incomplete right eye closure, and slight mouth movement on the right side (Figures 11.1, 11.2).

Palpation verification (PaVe)

Given the type of presentation/symptoms, palpation followed the Fascial Manipulation® for Internal Dysfunctions (FMID) protocol. This type of assessment takes into account the tensile structures for the head and neck region and their potential role in abnormal neural tension.

Assessment was essentially palpatory and was directed initially at the segments of caput (cp) and collum (cl) and, subsequently, the upper limb, including palpation of the proximal pivot points associated with the scapular (sc)

segment, and the distal tensors associated with the wrist (ca) segment. Palpatory assessment was also made of the superficial fascia of the head and neck. Upon palpation, no densification was identified in the distal tensors but there were multiple points identified in centers of coordination and centers of fusion in the fascia of the head and neck. The most densified points were found on the fascia of the right sternocleidomastoid (an-cl, an-la-cl, la-cl, ir-cl), right and left masseter (an-la-cp 3, la-cp 3, ir-cp 3), right and left temporalis (an-la-cp1, er-cp 2, la-cp 2), right posterior auricularis (er-cp 3), right scalenes (an-la-sc 1, 2), and right upper trapezius (la-sc). Densification was also found in the SMAS on the right side.

No specific distal tensor was identified in the wrist segments, but there appeared to be a prevalence of densification in points along the an-la diagonal and the lateral sequence on the frontal plane. Based on the degree of densification, as perceived by the therapist, the treatment

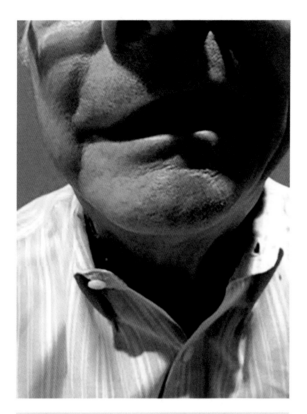

Figure 11.1
Before treatment: inability to raise the right upper lip

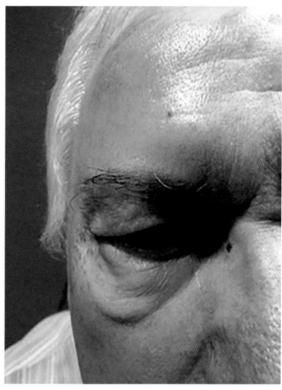

Figure 11.2
Before treatment: inability to close eye or raise brow

proceeded with the points where sliding was reduced the most and the tissue felt thickened and granular.

Treatment

1st treatment

The first treatment was directed towards the deep fascia, including centers of coordination (CC) on the frontal plane with the addition of two centers of fusion (CF) (Table 11.2).

2nd treatment

Patient follow-up was 1 week later. Upon re-assessment R. V. demonstrated improved motor function, but there was no change in drooling while taking a drink. Figures 11.3, 11.4 show the change in motor function.

Treatment on the second visit more specifically addressed the superficial fascia. It should be noted that, when recording superficial fascia treatment, each specific quadrant is indicated by the letter 'q' to distinguish it from a center of fusion (Table 11.3).

3rd treatment

Due to scheduling conflicts and patient holiday, R. V. was followed for a third assessment and treatment 3 weeks later.

The patient reported better overall mobility and sensation in the face, noting limited – if any – drooling while drinking. At this point, he was now grade II on the House–Brackmann facial nerve grading scale. His presentation upon arrival is seen in Figures 11.5, 11.6, 11.7,

Treatment of Bell's palsy
Larry Steinbeck

Table 11.2 1st Treatment					
Points treated	la-cp 3 rt	an-la-cl rt	an-la-cp 3 rt	la-cl rt	la-cp 2 lt

Table 11.3 2nd Treatment					
Points and quadrants	an-la-cp 1 rt	er-cp 3 rt	q an-la-cl rt	q re-la-cl lt	q an-la-cp

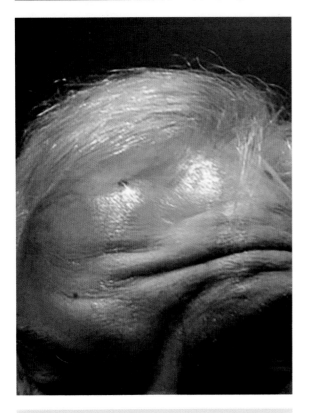

Figure 11.3
After first FM treatment: able to furl brow

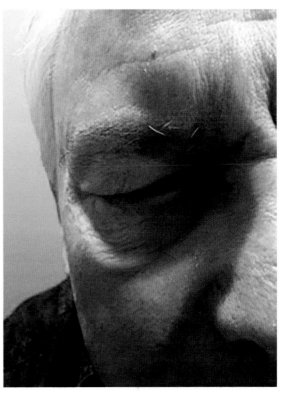

Figure 11.4
After first FM treatment: improved eye closing

where a 'grossly slight weakness is noticeable and possible slight synkinesis,' at rest 'normal resting tone and symmetry,' motion with 'forehead moderate to good function with the eye closing using minimum effort,' and 'slight asymmetry' in the mouth.

The patient felt encouraged by the changes that had occurred but was more surprised by comments from family and friends who noted a significant change in his facial expressions.

Treatment on this third visit is shown in Table 11.4.

Table 11.4 3rd Treatment				
Points and quadrants treated	ir-cp1 rt	me-cp1 rt	an-cp1 rt	re-la-cp1
	q re-la-cp1 rt	q re-me-cp1 rt	q an-me-cp2,3 rt	

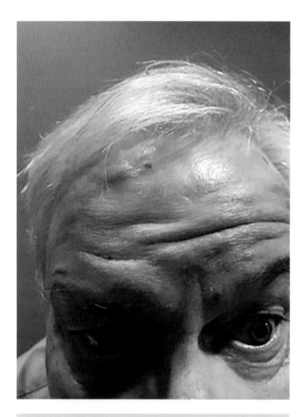

Figure 11.5
Further improvement in ability to furl brow

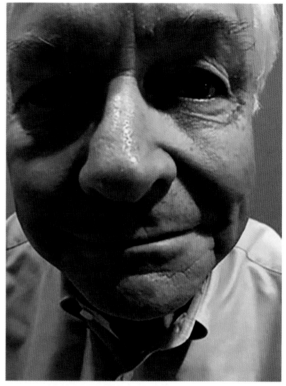

Figure 11.6
Improved smile, able to close mouth for drinking

Results

At this point, no further treatment was provided. Three weeks later the patient returned for some follow-up photographs. No significant gains were observed. The patient remained at grade II on the House–Brackmann scale for the facial nerve. Grade I on this scale is described as 'normal facial function in all areas.'

Discussion

This patient made significant visible changes in motor function along with significant change in functional tasks. Initially, he did not have adequate eye closure or the ability to seal his lips while drinking, but by the completion of treatment he was able to carry out these functions. This overall improvement in motor function permitted adequate hydration and lubrication of the cornea, as well as normalizing his ability to drink without drooling.

In journal articles regarding Bell's palsy (Eviston et al. 2015; Phan et al. 2016) there is some consensus that the injury to the facial nerve is due to a virus. In most instances, nerve and motor function return spontaneously within a few days or it is treated effectively with corticosteroids and/or antiviral medication. In this case, no improvement had been seen after 5 months and several different medications.

It was hypothesized that there could have been a densification that developed as a result of the infection to the facial nerve, affecting both the deep and superficial

Treatment of Bell's palsy

Larry Steinbeck

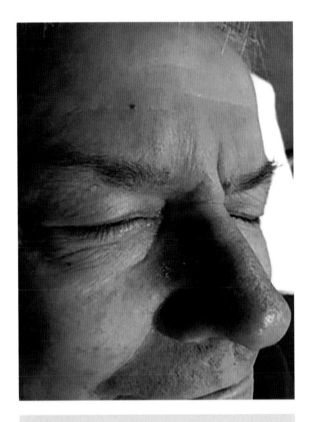

Figure 11.7
Able to close eye completely

fascia. In particular, the superficial fascia of the face envelops and connects all the mimic muscles, creating an organized fibrous, muscular network, while the deep fascia envelops the masticatory muscles, including the temporalis and masseter, and the salivary glands. Given that all muscles involved in chewing and swallowing are interconnected by fasciae, a normal tensional relationship in this fascial network is essential for correct function (Stecco C. 2015).

One reason for densification could have been the immobilization of the facial muscles consequent to the infection of the facial nerve and resultant paralysis. Raghavan et al. (2016) indicate that paralysis and immobility due to central nervous system injury lead to an increased volume of the extracellular matrix (ECM) surrounding the

neurovascular tissues. Presumably, a similar increase in ECM could also occur with paralysis and immobility due to peripheral nerve injury. Pavan et al. (2014) point out that viscosity of the ECM increases 'considerably with increasing distance between two surfaces' as reported in the above paper. One primary constituent of the ECM is hyaluronan (HA), which is an anionic, non-sulfated glycosaminoglycan distributed widely throughout connective, epithelial, and neural tissues, and it plays a role in determining ECM viscoelasticity as well as fibrosis development through signaling pathways (Albeiroti et al. 2015). Cowman et al. (2015) also discuss the role of HA in tissue stiffness. They state that manual intervention through deep friction manipulation may be effective via its shear rate, which alters the HA and ECM properties and, hence, the viscoelasticity in the surrounding tissue. Manual manipulation may produce a similar effect to hyaluronidases, which are enzymes that catabolize HA (Stern & Jedrzejas 2006).

In their book *Fascial Manipulation for Internal Dysfunction: Practical Part* (2016) Luigi and Antonio Stecco provide detail of the relationship between the superficial fascia and the deep fascia. Throughout the body, there are numerous vertical 'skin ligaments' that connect the hypodermis, the superficial fascia, and the deep fascia. They describe how these are not actual 'ligaments' since there is no bone to bone attachment. Instead, they should correctly be referred to as retinacula cutis superficialis, which connect the hypodermis and the superficial fascia, and the retinacula cutis profundus, which connect the superficial fascia to the deep fascia. These retinacula limit the degree of mobility between each layer with respect to the adjacent layer. They note that there are locations within the body where specialized aspects of the retinacula cutis permit firmer anchorage of the skin to the deep fascia. For example, you can easily identify a longitudinal specialization over the ligamentum nuchae that continues onto the occiput, and horizontally you can easily see a similar formation in the suboccipital region. They discuss how this organization of longitudinal and horizontal specialized reinforcements essentially divides the superficial fascia into quadrants. These quadrants can be demonstrated in the head, trunk, and limbs. In the second treatment reported in this case study, attention was directed towards the superficial fascia and in those instances a 'q' was used to identify the quadrant in which the superficial fascia was manipulated.

Densification of the fascia may have resulted in continued dysfunction of the fascial nerve by preventing telescoping at points of entry through the deep and superficial fascia. A clinical anatomy study on the musculocutaneous nerve (Macchi et al. 2007) states that 'the arrangement of the fibroadipose tissue sheaths may be compared to a "telescope" and may allow compliance between variations of length of the coracobrachialis muscle and the constant course of the musculocutaneous nerve.' The authors further state that this arrangement may explain the low frequency of entrapment syndrome involving the musculocutaneous nerve, which generally originates from physical activity or violent passive movements of the arm and forearm.

L. Stecco and A. Stecco (2016) also identify specific anatomical locations that can be considered points where fascia may cause potential nerve entrapment. These locations are described as:

- at the nerve root
- the nerve's passage through the deep fascia
- the nerve's passage within, as well as its exit from, the superficial fascia. In particular, after emerging from the stylomastoid foramen, the facial nerve gives rise to the posterior auricular branch. The facial nerve then passes through the parotid gland, which it does not innervate, to form the parotid plexus. Apart from the motor component originating from the parotid plexus, including five branches innervating the muscles of facial expression, the facial nerve has motor fibers for the mimic muscles comprised within the superficial fascia (Benninghoff & Goerttler 1986). The motor component could be affected by densification of the fascial tissue at any or all of these points.

Clinically, peripheral motor changes have been observed following decompression surgery on the spine (Watanabe et al. 2005; Macki et al. 2016) and a retrospective review of 12 patients who underwent decompression surgery for Bell's palsy, 21–70 days after onset, compared to 22 patients who had steroid and antiviral therapy without decompression concluded that final recovery rate did not differ significantly in the two groups; however, all patients in the decompression group recovered to at least House–Brackmann grade III at final follow-up (Kim et al. 2016).

In the case study presented in this chapter, we saw changes in motor function when addressing the points of passage of the facial nerve through the deep fascia (in particular: an-la-cl and ir-cp 3), and its association with the superficial fascia (q an-la-cp, q re-la-cp, q re-me-cp and q re-me-cp). The resolution of densification brought about by the treatment of both the deep and superficial fascia may have been similar to decompression on the nerve at multiple sites. Even though the nerve function may have been initially impaired by a virus, the delay in return may have been compounded by compression on the neural component from densification of the fascia as the nerve passes along its course. Essentially this may be ultimately due to immobilization associated with the initial nerve inhibition.

Conclusion

In these instances, where densification and alteration of the fascia coincide with changes in motor function, manipulation of the fascia may be useful in restoring motor function. When addressing dysfunctions of the 'neuromyofascial skeletal biomechanical system' the inclusion of treatment for both the deep and superficial fascia could introduce significant improvement in chronic peripheral nerve entrapment sequelae.

Treatment of Bell's palsy
Larry Steinbeck

References

Albeiroti S, Soroosh A and de la Motte CA (2015) Hyaluronan's role in fibrosis: A pathogenic factor or a passive player? BioMed Research International 2015:790203. doi: 10.1155/2015/790203.

Benninghoff A and Goerttler K (1986) Trattato di anatomia umana. Padua: Piccin.

Cowman M, Schmidt TA, Raghavan P and Stecco A (2015) Viscoelastic properties of hyaluronan in physiological conditions. F1000 Research 4 622. doi: 10.12688/f1000research.6885.1.

de Almeida JR, Guyatt GH, Sud S, Dorion J, Hill MD et al. (2014) Management of Bell palsy: Clinical guidelines. Canadian Medical Association Journal 186 (12) 917–22.

Eviston TJ, Croxson GR, Kennedy PG, Hadlock T and Krishnan AV (2015) Bell's palsy: Aetiology, clinical features, and multidisciplinary care. Journal of Neourology, Neurosurgery, and Psychiatry 86 1356–61.

Kim SH, Jung J, Lee JH, Byun JY, Park MS and Yeo SG (2016) Delayed facial nerve decompression for Bell's palsy. European Archives of Oto-rhino-laryngology 273 (7) 1755–60.

Macchi, V, Tiengo C, Porzionato A, Parenti A, Stecco C, Bassetto F, Scapinelli R, Taglialavoro G and De Caro R (2007) Musculocutaneous nerve: Histotopographic study and clinical implications. Clinical Anatomy 20 400–6.

Macki M, Syeda S, Kerezoudis P, Gokaslan ZL, Bydon A and Bydon M (2016) Preoperative motor strength and time to surgery are the most important predictors of improvement in foot drop due to degenerative lumbar disease. Journal of the Neurological Sciences 361 133–6.

Pahn NT, Panizza B and Wallwork B (2016) A general practice approach to Bell's palsy. Australian Family Physician 11, 794–7.

Pavan PG, Stecco A, Stern R and Stecco C (2014) Painful connections: Densification versus fibrosis of fascia. Current Pain and Headache Reports 18 (8) 441. doi: 10.1007/s11916-014-0441-4.

Raghavan P, Lu Y, Mirchandani M and Stecco A (2016) Human recombinant hyaluronidase injections for upper limb muscle stiffness in individuals with cerebral injury: A case series. EBioMedicine 9 306–13.

Stecco C (2015) Functional atlas of the human fascial system. Edinburgh: Churchill Livingstone, Elsevier.

Stecco L and Stecco A (2016) Fascial manipulation for internal dysfunctions: Practical part. Padua: Piccin.

Stern R and Jedrzejas MJ (2006) Hyaluronidases: Their genomics, structures, and mechanisms of action. Chemical Reviews 106 (3) 818–39.

Sun MZ, Oh MC, Safaee M, Kaur G and Parsa AT (2012) Neuroanatomical correlation of the House–Brackmann grading system in the microsurgical treatment of vestibular schwannoma. Neurosurgical Focus 33 (3) E7. doi: 10.3171/2012.6.

Watanabe K, Hasegawa K, Hirano T, Endo N, Yamazaki A and Homma T (2005) Anterior spinal decompression and fusion for cervical flexion myelopathy in young patients. Journal of Neurosurgery. Spine 3 (2) 86–91.

Fascial Manipulation® for Internal Dysfunction (FMID) in the management of post-partum urinary incontinence in a runner

Colleen Whiteford, USA

EDITOR'S COMMENT

This chapter presents a case report involving post-partum urinary incontinence in a mother of two children who had been forced to abandon running due to her disturbance. After five treatments of Fascial Manipulation for Internal Dysfunction (FMID), plus two sessions addressing running analysis and exercises, she was literally up and running again. The author of this chapter is specialized in orthopedics and dry needling and has been working with the Fascial Manipulation®–Stecco® method since 2014, 30 years after she first graduated as a physical therapist. She explains how this method provides a system that guides her in determining the most effective sites for intervention yet, at the same time, encompasses her knowledge and experience regarding evaluation and treatment. In addition, the author suggests that while fascia is not often considered in the management of many diagnoses, including urinary incontinence, the fascial system has the potential to be very influential by virtue of its extensive anatomy.

Author's background

I am a 1984 physical therapy graduate of Saint Louis University in St Louis, Missouri (USA). In 1986 I co-founded Appalachian Physical Therapy with my physical therapist husband, Bill, and continue in full-time clinical practice with our three offices in Virginia and North Carolina (USA). I received board certification as an orthopedic specialist in 2009 from the American Board of Physical Therapy Specialties, and also a Doctor of Physical Therapy degree from Shenandoah University in Winchester, Virginia, in 2011. I became certified in dry needling

through Myopain Seminars® in 2010, and later joined the faculty assisting with teaching needling courses. I began working with Fascial Manipulation® (FM) in 2014, and have since completed Levels I, II, and III and also presented on the subject at numerous local, state, and national events.

Experience with Fascial Manipulation®–Stecco® method

The pursuit of specialist certification was fueled by my motivation to be practicing at the highest level of my profession, accomplishing better clinical results. My practice model of joint and soft tissue mobilization, exercise, education, dry needling, and other modalities served patients well and distinguished our practice. Even so, some patients would experience improvement but not resolution. Others seemed to have a full recovery but would return later with the same issue or a new complaint. Many presented with multiple and seemingly unrelated problems, which were often overwhelming and frustrating.

I was exposed to the FM model in 2014 at an introductory course. As I listened to the instructor expound on the chemical milieu found in a fascial densification I was struck by the similarity it bore to the science of myofascial trigger points. The weekend experience impressed me enough to register for the follow-up Level I FM course, which was canceled due to lack of participants. Seeking more training, I purchased the practical text and tried to apply the system myself. Even with my minimal training in the model, I recognized a positive change in outcomes with patients in terms of response, sustainability of improvement, and the ability to address widespread multiple issues. I convinced my coworkers of the value of the approach and arranged for private Level I and II courses in our clinics. Since then we have all been utilizing FM daily on practically every patient we see, with remarkable results. FM has become the fundamental element of our practice model.

In an odd way, FM has not really changed how I practice, yet at the same time turned it upside down. I continue to compile a patient history but search for different elements such as past problems, extremity cramping, and recurrent complaints. Training in Level III has equipped me to ask about constipation, reflux, and a host of other maladies I once relegated to the sphere of medicine. I now have a framework for understanding how these issues relate to the apparent musculoskeletal complaints driving patients to my practice. I still visually inspect patients, but I now have a plausible explanation and approach for addressing their musculoskeletal deformities. I continue to meticulously assess movement for quantity and quality. But instead of focusing exclusively and microscopically on where it is limited, dysfunctional, painful, or weak, I am now able to put it into the much broader context of how it relates to the rest of the body and the individual's other problems. In many cases, this leads me to work in body segments very remote to the area of the primary complaint.

I still use manual therapy, especially soft tissue mobilization. With FM I have a system of evaluation and treatment that guides me to determine the most effective sites for intervention. The FM model has not driven me to abandon all I have learned in my years of training and practice. Rather, it encompasses my knowledge and experience regarding evaluation and treatment, expands it to include a total body perspective, and organizes it in a way that can be practically implemented for each patient encounter. Ultimately, the results have been a substantial and sustainable improvement in primary complaints as well as seemingly unrelated issues; expedited response time in fewer visits; and patient/client satisfaction that is only rivaled by this therapist's own satisfaction. I believe I have finally accomplished my goal of practicing at the highest level of my profession.

The American Physical Therapy Association, in its vision statement, charges me and my colleagues to 'Transform society by optimizing movement to improve the human experience' (see www.apta.org). At Shenandoah University, Winchester (VA), in 2014, Dr Shirley Sahrmann identified the musculoskeletal, neurological, integumentary, and respiratory systems as integral parts of the movement system. By the same line of reasoning, the urinary, digestive, reproductive, circulatory, lymphatic, metabolic, endocrine, and sensory components of the human body should also be considered as components of the movement system. Leaders in our association propose embracing 'regional interdependence,' which is the perspective that pain and dysfunction may be arising from tissues remote but related to the site of complaint (Wainner et al. 2007). While we may agree that these concepts are admirable, they remain hypothetical constructs unless they are accompanied by a practical way to incorporate them into everyday evaluation and treatment. In my years of clinical practice, specialty training, and continuing education I have never encountered an approach that aided me in implementing these ideas so comprehensively and successfully in practice as I have with FM.

CASE REPORT

Fascial Manipulation® for Internal Dysfunction in the management of post-partum urinary incontinence in a runner

Introduction

E. B. is a 34-year-old mother of two, ages 4 and 7. The first child was delivered by Cesarean section, and the second by a very difficult vaginal delivery. After recovery from the second, she returned to running but quickly developed diastasis recti (DR) as well as stress urinary incontinence (UI). The UI manifested when running, jumping on a trampoline with her children, and sneezing. She continued to try the trampoline, but would tell her children she had to stop because 'Mommy just peed her pants.' She also abandoned running.

Wanting to be active, she sought help from a women's health physical therapist 1 year after the onset of symptoms. Treatments included Kegels, breathing retraining, and core stabilization with emphasis on the transversus abdominis and pelvic floor elevation. She reportedly worked diligently, relating that her therapist commented on the excellent chart she kept outlining her performance. An internal pelvic examination was performed with the therapist determining that she had 'adequate pelvic floor strength,' and no further internal work was performed. After 5 weeks with five visits, she felt that her DR might be improved, but her UI was unchanged. Her therapist encouraged her to try running but UI persisted and she discontinued care.

E. B. explored exercise programs she could find on the internet but had no success altering the UI. A physical therapist family member suggested further physical therapy and located our facility on the internet. E. B. read about our programs and presented for evaluation and treatment under direct access without a physician referral.

At the time of her initial evaluation, E. B. related an additional history that included hypermobility, headaches, a hemorrhoid, ankle sprains, shin splints, and knee pain. She rated a numeric pain scale (NPS) as 0, citing a 'weak core and pelvic floor' as her only complaints. With a second outcome measure, the Patient Specific Functional Scale (PSFS), due to the UI she rated herself at 2/10 or 80% disability with running, jumping on the trampoline, and doing jumping jacks. Ankle sprains and shin splints with running were cited as her oldest problems, dating back to high school, with headaches beginning later in college. She also reported the recent development of morning lower back pain in the coccyx region. This seemed worse with prolonged sitting and improved with movement.

Hypothesis

In the FM model, history is critical in the clinical reasoning process with segments of oldest complaint meriting attention. Since her primary complaint of UI involved the pelvic region and the oldest segment of dysfunction was the ankles, these areas were hypothesized as influencing her complaints. In the FM model, UI is classified as an internal dysfunction (ID) and she was therefore approached from an FMID perspective. Multiple comments from her associating UI with the closure of the DR prompted a discussion that while both reflected a problem with a tensile structure, the two issues were not necessarily co-dependent since they can exist in isolation. As her DR was improved from the onset and was not as disruptive as the UI, the remainder of care centered on UI.

Methodology

An inspection revealed a healthy body mass with no obvious structural deformities of the trunk, lower extremities, or feet. Gait demonstrated no abnormalities.

Movement verification (MoVe)

The next step in the FM system is mobility assessment, termed movement verification (MoVe). The pelvic (pv) segment lacks freedom of movement compared to the lumbar (lu) segment, and lu was therefore selected for MoVe (Table 12.1). Based on her history, the ankles/talus (ta) bilaterally were also selected for MoVe. Hypermobility was apparent, potentially disguising mobility

Table 12.1 Movement verification (MoVe) for the patient assessing triplanar mobility in the lumbar and talus segments. Genu segment was later added in with a global MoVe using a squat

Movement verification (MoVe)			
	Sagittal plane	Frontal plane	Horizontal plane
Lumbar (lu): trunk forward bend (FB), backward bend (BB), side bend (SB)	Hypermobility, trunk forward bend palming floor. Backward bend restricted and sore low back	Trunk side bend full bilaterally	Trunk rotation left mildly limited. Full right
Ankle/talus (ta): ankle dorsi-flexion (DF), plantar flexion (FB), inversion, eversion	Walking on heels and forefeet normal bilaterally	Walking on lateral and medial borders of feet normal bilaterally	Not tested
Knee/genu (ge)	Global MoVe: squat. Full, mild crepitus, sore right knee		

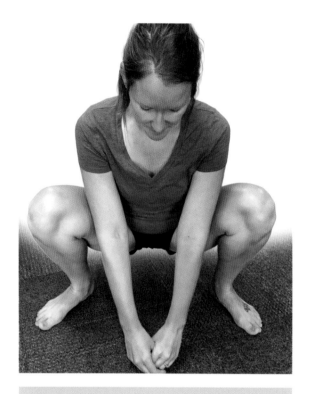

Figure 12.1
Patient performing a squat, which is considered to be a comprehensive or global movement test for the genu segment

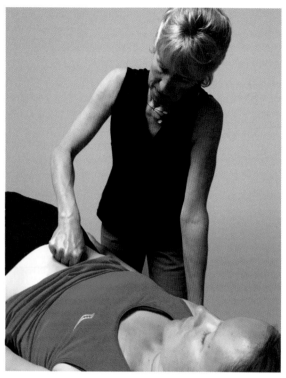

Figure 12.2
Therapist palpating ante-medio-lumbi 2, a principal center of fusion in the lumbar segment for the anteroposterior internal fascial sequence

abnormalities, but deficits with some movements were evident. Since the knees were identified in her history, a global MoVe test for the knees was added with a squat (Figure 12.1). While there is much debate in the literature over the ideal mechanics of a squat, this practitioner has found that it is clinically simple and efficient to allow the subject to perform the maneuver in whatever manner they choose (heels up or down, arms flexed or at the sides, lumbar lordosis or flat). Characteristics of the squat, such as fullness of movement, difficulty, pain reports, and crepitus are noted for future comparison.

Palpation verification (PaVe)

The next element in the evaluation, according to the FM model, was palpation verification (PaVe). The patient

was first educated as to fascia, the sliding system, and the densification hypothesis. She was positioned supine and palpation was performed in the lu, pv, and ta segments following the guidelines of FMID. This consisted of palpating the principal centers of fusion (CF) in the lumbar segment, namely an-me-lu 2 (Figure 12.2), an-la-lu 2, and ir-lu bilaterally, in an effort to identify the most densified points based on the examiner's perception and the patient's report. Palpation was continued into the pv segment with an-me-pv 2, an-la-pv 2, and ir-pv p bilaterally. Next, the CFs of ta were palpated bilaterally in an effort to identify a distal tensor. With none being found there, palpation was continued to the feet, with an-me-pe 1 bilaterally presenting as densified and painful. Based on the patient's report as well as the examiner's perception of the most densified CFs, the antero-posterior (AP) internal fascia sequence was identified as the most involved. This sequence includes the ante-medio and retro-medio catenaries. A DR of 1.5 finger widths was also identified, which she stated had not changed for the past 2 years.

Treatment

Findings of the evaluation were discussed with the patient. With her consent treatment was begun using FM to the most densified sites (Table 12.2):

1. Post-treatment MoVe demonstrated increased lumbar extension without low back discomfort. She was instructed in a version of a posterior pelvic tilt exercise with simultaneous blowing up of a balloon (Postural Restoration® Institute), an exercise she noted was similar to ones she had worked with in the past. She was also advised that changes in bladder function might not be immediately evident.

2. Five days later E. B. returned for her second visit thrilled with her improvement. She reported feeling like 'her bladder was in a different place.' She had been able to jump on the trampoline and sneeze without any urine leakage. She even tried running for less than 10 minutes and did not have leakage, but did experience right knee pain. She also noted her back pain and hemorrhoid were better. MoVe revealed lumbar extension and rotation left were mildly restricted. Treatment was continued with FMID in supine in

the AP line due to her favorable response to her first visit. PaVe was also performed in prone for assessment of lu, pv, and the hips (cx) as these are key segments associated with UI. Densification was found in the CC of er-lu rt and this was treated with FM, as well as other sites. Further education was provided on hypermobility. As she was anxious to be doing some form of exercise and had a therapy exercise ball and hula hoop at home, she was begun with seated triplanar pelvic ball exercises and standing hula hoop activities, which she enjoyed doing with her children.

3. Anxious to resume running, she returned 2 days later for a session with another therapist specializing in athletes. She was continuing to do well with no leakage while jumping on the trampoline, sneezing, or running in the yard playing with her children. No FM was performed on this visit, and she received a running analysis, recommendations on returning to running, shoe assessment and education, and instruction in additional exercises.

4. E. B. returned for her fourth visit 5 days after the running analysis with new shoes. She had worked up to a 30-minute run/walk combination and did not have any urine leakage, knee, or back pain. She reported that since her last FM session her right knee symptoms had changed, and she now had discomfort in the right knee with sitting on her feet (Figure 12.3). Assumption of this position reproduced her right knee

Table 12.2 Centers of coordination (CC) and centers of fusion (CF) treated on patient throughout the course of her care				
Treatment				
Visit 1	an–me–pv 2 lt	an–me–pv 3 rt	an–me–pe 1 bi		
Visit 2	an–me–cx lt	an–me–ge 3 rt	an–pe lt	ir–ge rt	er–lu rt
Visit 3	Running analysis, shoe education, exercise				
Visit 4	re–me–ge 1 bi	er–ge bi			
Visit 5	an–me–cp 2 rt	ir–cp 2 lt	er–cp 3 rt		
Visit 6	Running analysis, education, exercise				
Visit 7	re–me–cp 3 lt	re–me–sc lt	re–me–pe 1 & 2 bi	an–me–lu 1 rt	

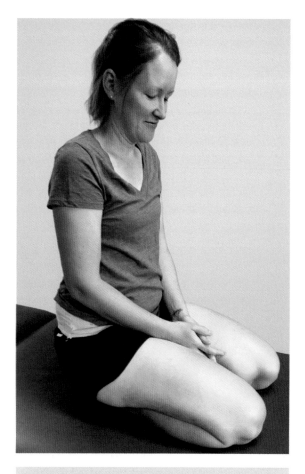

Figure 12.3
At her fourth visit the patient reported discomfort in the right knee with sitting on her feet. As assumption of this position reproduced her right knee symptoms it was considered her 'personalized' movement verification for assessment post-treatment

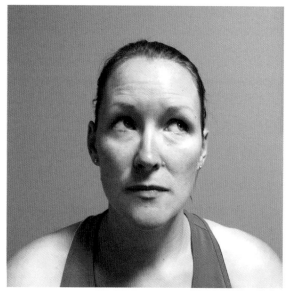

Figure 12.4
At her fifth visit, the patient presented with a headache. Given that her history included headaches, movement verification in the head (caput: cp) was performed, with superior/lateral movement of the eyes to the left exacerbating her headache

symptoms, and this was considered her MoVe for assessment post-treatment. Her squat was full but sore in the right knee with crepitus. PaVe revealed densifications in the thighs and knees posteriorly and these were addressed with FM. Post-treatment she had full resolution of knee symptoms with squatting and sitting on her feet, although crepitus persisted.

5. E. B. was seen 1 week later, reporting increasing time running without knee pain or UI. The day after her last treatment she developed a migraine headache without typical triggers (lack of sleep, weather, pollen, certain foods). Mild right knee discomfort was present with sitting on her feet, and she currently presented with a headache. Recalling that her history included headaches, MoVe in the head (caput: cp) was performed, with superior/lateral movement of the eyes to the left exacerbating her headache (Figure 12.4). FM was continued with a focus on the head, after which there was an immediate improvement in her headache.

6. Two days later E. B. returned for further running analysis, education, and assistance with her exercises from the consulting athletic therapist.

She was successfully increasing her running time and distance with no UI. Her headache was completely resolved. No FM was performed.

7. One week after her previous FM session E. B. returned for her final visit. She was excited to be increasing running gradually to avoid injury but not limited by UI. She was successfully jumping on the trampoline for 15 minutes limited by fatigue but not bladder leakage. Her right knee was mildly symptomatic when sitting on her feet for an extended period. She reported mild lower back tightness with lumbar extension, and she had experienced one mild headache since last treated. MoVe demonstrated minimal lower back tightness in extension, mild right knee discomfort with sitting on her feet and trace soreness behind the left eye with superior/lateral movements of the eyes. She was treated with FM to the most densified sites identified with palpation. The feet (pe) were extremely involved as manifested by the extended time it took to accomplish tissue glide here as well as her reports of extreme discomfort during treatment. This was not surprising considering the chronicity of her lower extremity running injuries. MoVe post-treatment demonstrated full resolution of her low back, knee and head symptoms. The PSFS was scored at 9/10 or 10% disability. She was encouraged to continue gradually building up her mileage, and no further appointments were scheduled. In a follow-up assessment via phone 1 month after discharge she reported to be doing very well with no UI, and was continuing to increase her running time while training for a 10-kilometer run. She also reported she was not being compliant with her home exercise program.

Discussion

In the United States, UI is typically relegated to the scope of women's health physical therapists possessing skills and training in internal pelvic examination and treatment. This supports a culture where UI is addressed as a specialty area of practice. Conversely, therapists not trained in internal pelvic techniques may consider the pelvic region, and diagnoses such as UI, to be mutually exclusive from other diagnoses a patient may manifest. Yet the evidence supports that these issues can be interrelated and should be considered as such (Cassidy et al. 2017). In their literature review of 41 scientific publications, Ramin et al. (2016) highlighted a strong functional and anatomical relationship linking the fascia of the low back, abdomen, and pelvic floor. Many approaches in the treatment of UI emphasize the role of pelvic floor muscle activity as the problem, and normalization of such muscle activity as the solution, be it facilitation or inhibition. Kurz and Borello-France (2017) advocate considering sources beyond the pelvic floor muscles, such as the hip, and the influence movement impairments of these joints may have on the pelvic floor musculature. Overall, these traditional approaches incorporating multimodal aspects of education, breathing retraining, exercise, biofeedback, and muscle facilitation/inhibition have been shown to yield some benefit. Yet they often rely on multiple treatment sessions, internal examination, an extended time period to accomplish results, specialized training, in some cases specialized equipment, and prolonged compliance with home exercises which patients are known to abandon (Borrello-France et al. 2008).

This case report demonstrates a favorable response for a patient using FM methodology. Although fascia is not often considered in the management of many diagnoses, including UI, the fascial system has the potential to be very influential by virtue of its expansive anatomy and relationship to the internal organs and musculoskeletal system (Stecco C. 2015). Fascia also possesses the capability to transmit force between remote body segments (Stecco C. 2015). L. Stecco and C. Stecco (2014) liken the trunk to a tensile structure with catenaries or extensions, represented by the limbs. Abnormal tension, such as a fascial densification might produce at any point along the structure, has the potential to disrupt normal movement and function. The fasciae of the pelvic diaphragm are especially subject to influence from the lower extremities (Stecco L. & Stecco C. 2014). In the case of E. B., it was hypothesized that injuries to the ankles initiated her problems. Issues with shin splints and knee pain indicated unresolved dysfunction, possibly reflecting a loss of normal slide between tissue interfaces of the deep fascia in the lower extremities. This was confirmed by the intensity of her discomfort when FM was administered to her feet – the segment harboring her oldest problem. Further tissue overload was introduced to the system during her second pregnancy and delivery, which tensioned the system beyond its capacity to compensate, resulting in a DR and UI. With her first course of therapy, the patient underwent an internal pelvic examination that reportedly did not demonstrate muscle dysfunction or weakness. She was treated in a traditional manner using exercises which, interestingly enough, included pelvic floor elements. Despite her admirable and atypical compliance with her program, she experienced no change in UI. While she reported improvement in the DR, one might argue that it was ensuing regardless of her efforts (Kurz & Borello-France 2017).

Conclusion

The course of this patient's care in the management of UI using FM is noteworthy for several reasons:

1. She experienced a significant change in UI after one visit.

2. Her course of care was complete in 30 days, with five visits using FM and two visits for running analysis and exercise.

3. No internal pelvic examination or treatment was utilized.

4. No special equipment was utilized.

5. Her primary physical therapist had minimal training in traditional women's health care.

6. Secondary complaints of headaches and lower extremity symptoms were incorporated into her program with improvement.

7. The patient remained fully continent at a one-month phone follow-up.

8. Sustained changes in her UI were not dependent on her compliance with exercises.

The staggering impact of UI burdens people worldwide from a financial and quality of life perspective (Zhu et al. 2009). While much time, money, and effort are expended by patients and practitioners in attempts to eradicate this problem, it persists at an alarming and disheartening level. Perhaps this is due, in part, to a lack of attention to fascia and its potential for influencing UI. Many conditions treated, at least from this practitioner's experience, could be prevented or minimized with earlier intervention than is typically administered. In the case of E. B., one can only speculate regarding the impact this relatively early intervention and resolution of UI may have throughout her lifespan. One might even question whether she could have avoided the UI and DR if FM had been utilized prior to her pregnancies. The FM system offers a viable option for assessing and treating those with similar complaints.

FMID in the management of post-partum urinary incontinence in a runner
Colleen Whiteford

References

Borello-France D, Downey P, Zyczynski H and Raus C (2008) Continence and quality-of-life outcomes 6 months following an intensive pelvic-floor muscle exercise program for female stress urinary incontinence: A randomized trial comparing low- and high-frequency maintenance exercise. Physical Therapy 88 (12) 1545–53.

Cassidy T, Fortin A, Kaczmer S, Shumaker J and Szeto J (2017) Relationship between back pain and urinary incontinence in the Canadian population. Physical Therapy 97 (4) 449–54.

Kurz J and Borello-France D (2017) Movement system impairment-guided approach to the physical therapist treatment of a patient with postpartum pelvic organ prolapse and mixed urinary incontinence: Case report. Physical Therapy 97 (4) 464–77.

Ramin A, Macchi V, PoRzionato A, De Caro R and Stecco C (2016) Fascial continuity of the pelvic floor with the abdominal and lumbar region. Pelviperineology [e-journal] 35 (1) 3–6. Available: http://www.pelviperineology.org/march-2016/pdf/pelviperineology-march-2016-hd.pdf> [17 December 2017].

Stecco C (2015) Functional atlas of the human fascial system. Edinburgh: Churchill Livingstone, Elsevier.

Stecco L and Stecco C (2014) Fascial manipulation for internal dysfunctions. Padua: Piccin.

Wainner R, Whitman J, Cleland J and Flynn T (2007) Regional interdependence: A musculoskeletal examination model whose time has come. Journal of Orthopaedic and Sports Physical Therapy 37(11) 658–60.

Zhu L, Lang J, Liu C, Han S, Huang J and Li X (2009) The epidemiological study of women with urinary incontinence and risk factors for stress urinary incontinence in China. Menopause 16 (4) 831–6.

Section 3
Other perspectives

The three chapters in this section present other viewpoints regarding the application of the Fascial Manipulation®–Stecco® method. The first chapter introduces two valid hypotheses regarding variations that the author suggests practitioners of this method could be applying in their practice. The second chapter, a randomized clinical pilot study, is just one example of how selected parameters can be examined in detail and how the theoretical bases of this method offer different avenues for research. The final chapter examines the treatment of neurological pediatric cases, an area that is yet to be fully documented but which has exciting potential for preparation of movement training.

EDITOR'S COMMENT

It is a great honor to introduce this chapter by a renowned author in the field of chiropractic and, in particular, soft tissue treatment. This author, who introduced the Fascial Manipulation®-Stecco® met-hod to the USA in 2011, has an impressive curriculum that spans almost 60 years of intensive clinical practice, writing and teaching. Here he presents two plausible hypotheses that will surely spark debate amongst practitioners of this method in general. The first hypothesis introduces the concept of a functional versus a pathological point and suggests that therapists should be recognizing the difference between both types and including them in their analysis and treatment. This hypothesis is substantiated by a case report. The second hypothesis addresses the possibility that certain lines of Stecco points may deserve more attention as compared to other lines. In particular, the author focuses on Stecco's retro-medio (re-me) diagonal line in which the multifidi are immersed, suggesting that it represents both a functional and pathological pathway that should be assessed and probably treated for back pain even though it may not have been identified as a primary altered structure during assessment.

Author's background

In chiropractic practice since 1960, I subsequently obtained a Master of Science degree and a diplomate in chiropractic orthopedics. Realizing the importance of soft tissue with respect to the treatment of joints I took many courses in soft tissue methods. Since 1985 I have lectured nationally and internationally on soft tissue. Some of the soft tissue methods taught were Cyriax's friction massage, strain/counterstrain, post facilitation stretch, myofascial release, muscle energy, Graston Technique®, Mattes' Active Isolated Stretching, Mulligan methods, Voyer's ELDOA™ (Longitudinal Osteo-Articular Decoaptation of the Spine) and others. I have authored and edited three editions of *Functional Soft-Tissue Examination and Treatment by Manual Methods* (1991, 1999, 2007) and more than 300 articles on soft tissue subjects, some of which have been peer-reviewed. In 2013 I became a certified Fascial Manipulation®–Stecco® method (FM) instructor. I invited Dr Antonio Stecco to the United States to teach FM in 2011, and the rest is history.

Introduction

This chapter discusses two new hypotheses that I have been utilizing for several years with outstanding results. They include the necessity of treating other than Stecco points to enhance FM results and the possibility that certain lines of Stecco points may deserve more importance when compared to other lines. Even though a patient might respond to treatment of a particular line, is it possible that another line relating pathologically to the patient's complaint should also be treated? Treatment of a related line, such as Stecco's retro-medio (re-me) diagonal in which the multifidi are immersed, might speed up recovery or even help prevent recidivism. Sometimes a particular line that did not appear noticeably densified may deserve our attention.

Luigi Stecco states in the introduction of a recent textbook (Stecco L. & Stecco A. 2017) that his early treatments were 'directed at the location of pain in the various joints.' He compared this method of treatment to Cyriax technique and stated that there were occasions when due to local inflammation he was unable to treat these areas. He eventually moved on to points in the surrounding areas that organized the activity of various muscles that moved the joint. Luigi Stecco believes that the site of pain or the center of perception (CP) is rarely the cause of pain but only a 'mere consequence of the dysfunction.' He states that the cause is the densification of the center of coordination

(CC) resulting in an uncoordinated activity of the muscular fibers. Except for some centers of fusion (CFs) that are located near a painful joint, most of the CFs are not directly on pathological tissue.

Hypothesis I

FM practitioners should recognize the difference between a functional and a pathological point and include both types in their analysis and treatment.

Have you ever experienced a case where you have used FM treatment for a problem, but weeks later or after several treatments, while the patient's pain had lessened, some functional tests were still painful? The patient may have been discharged or refused treatment without their problem completely resolved. I think most FM practitioners have experienced this type of situation. We determined that we treated the proper myofascial line or sequence and balanced the patient properly. After a number of FM treatments, we may have reached a point where the patient symptoms were no longer improving. At this stage, we might have reviewed the history to determine if there was an old injury that the patient failed to remember and possibly a silent point that we missed. Functional testing of the area had improved but remained painful and the patient did not make a complete recovery. Is it possible that restoring muscle coordination was not enough to complete the healing cycle?

By functional, FM relates principally to the restoration of peripheral motor coordination rather than direct tissue pathological change. Over time it is thought that restoring muscle coordination and alleviating pain should help restore pathological tissue to a more normal state. Functional rather than pathologic is also treated with the Fascial Manipulation Internal Dysfunction (FMID) approach. 'Functional disease refers to no serious observable change in the structure of an organ or its part' (Stecco L. & Stecco A. 2016).

A pathological point (PP) refers to a 'fibrosis-like problem similar to the process of scarring, with the deposition of excessive amounts of fibrotic connective tissue, reflective of a reparative or reactive process such as a tendinosis' (Pavan et al. 2014). Densification differs from pathology 'since there is no macroscopic alteration of the morphology of the fascia that would be seen on dissection or biopsy' (Stecco C 2015). A pathological point can be a fascial fibrosis or a chronic densification affecting the gliding between collagen fibrous bundles and within the fibrous layers rather than in loose connective tissue. These areas create local pain when tested and respond to deep friction massage primarily by causing a proliferation of fibroblasts (see below).

In FM, even though a resistive test, for example, shoulder external rotation may be painful, the final decision of where to treat in FM is based on the palpation of CCs/CFs along 10 fascial lines, whether over CCs of agonist and antagonist myofascial units, along unidirectional CCs of a myofascial sequence, or CFs located along diagonals or spirals. There is no question that FM procedure represents one of the great breakthroughs in the evolution of soft tissue treatment.

A pathological point, or PP, is located over pathologic tissue. Some common areas that may require local treatment could be:

- sprained acromioclavicular ligament
- knee or elbow collateral ligaments
- ankle ligamentous sprain
- rotator cuff insertions at the capsule
- musculotendinous areas
- gluteus medius insertions on the greater trochanter
- lateral or medial epicondyle
- spinal capsular facets
- areas in the ribcage

plus other sites in the upper and lower extremities. Often these areas may be diagnosed by magnetic resonance imaging (MRI) as insertional tendinosis of the gluteus medius, supraspinatus or infraspinatus tendon. The PP represents a chronic tissue alteration. Classic characteristics of 'tendinosis' include degenerative changes in the collagenous matrix, hypercellularity, hypervascularity, and a lack of inflammatory cells, which has challenged the original misnomer 'tendinitis' (Abate et al. 2009). Many tendonitis type conditions revert to a chronic tendinosis. Most PPs are located on muscles, ligaments, tendons and joint capsules proximal or distal to an FM point.

The selected FM myofascial lines may have been balanced by FM procedure, but the site of pain may still remain painful when stressed, allowing an unresolved result. This area might require a local treatment. Before Luigi Stecco discovered the fascial kinetic chain, local treatment had been a prime mode of treatment and still proves to be of value. Adding FM to restore coordination coupled with local treatment to actual tissue pathology allows a total healing solution. The question that this chapter will attempt to answer is: Where are some pathological points located and when should they be treated?

Treatment on PPs can be administered by transverse friction massage (Hammer 1991), similar to FM, except for the treatment time and location. A famous proponent of friction massage on the pathologic tissue was an English orthopedist, James Cyriax, MD (Ombregt et al. 2003). Cyriax recommended two 20-minute treatments a week usually for muscle areas, tendon insertions, and ligaments. Over the years his physical therapists limited their massage to around 10 minutes. For many of these PPs, he recommended treatment for over 'a month or more, effective in 6–10 sessions or not at all' (Lundon 2007). Today, the use of instrument-assisted soft tissue mobilization, laser, extracorporeal shock wave therapy, and other modalities over the PP may speed up the healing process and possibly may even speed up treatment on FM points.

Friction massage theories

There have been many hypotheses describing the benefits and use of friction massage. Some theories deal with connective tissue regeneration based on the stimulation and action of inflammatory cells, vascular and lymphatic endothelial

cells, and fibroblasts, beginning with the release of inflammatory mediators and ending with the remodeling of the repaired tissue (Lundon 2007). Fibroblastic proliferation is probably the most significant factor in healing since, when these cells are stimulated by manual pressure, they reproduce new extracellular matrix, including collagen, elastin, cytokines, and growth factors. Lundon (2007) further states that 'Fibroblastic proliferation and activation are key events in the healing process of connective tissue based structures and are responsible for gene expression and thereby production of cellular mediators of healing and synthesis of collagen.' A controlled animal study demonstrated an acceleration of ligament healing after surgically induced ligament injury using instrument-assisted soft tissue mobilization (Loghmani & Warden 2009). Recently, endocannabinoid receptors have been found in fascial tissue and concentrated in fibroblasts. It has been found that these receptors 'suppress pro-inflammatory cytokines such as IL-1 beta and TNF-alpha and increase anti-inflammatory cytokines' (Fede et al. 2016).

Pathological points vs FM points

Functional evaluation for pathological points are the standard orthopedic resistive and passive tests. For example, a patient with shoulder pain and weakness on resisted external rotation might lead to interpreting the infraspinatus tendon as the possible local pain generator. Pathological testing is meant to test the area of pain, palpate it, and treat. An FM practitioner would take note of the test but not necessarily incriminate the tissue taking part in shoulder external rotation. Conversely, if a practitioner is thinking about a pathological point he/she would immediately think of the tendinous area at the capsule where the infraspinatus inserts. If an FM examiner incriminated the CC of extrarotation-humerus (er-hu) as part of a sequence to be treated, the point location for er-hu would be just below the humeral head, over the posterior aspect of the deltoid. The pathologic point for resisted shoulder external rotation would be treated more proximally, on the infraspinatus tendon at the capsule (Figure 13.1). Friction over this PP should eventually produce a local anesthesia and resisted shoulder external rotation pain should improve. Ideally, FM procedure could be attempted first, but if after evaluation and

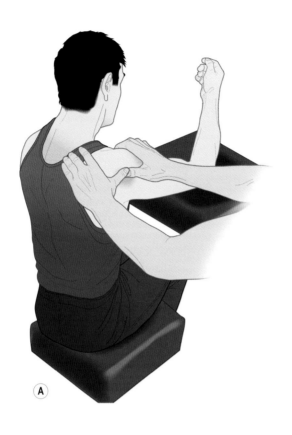

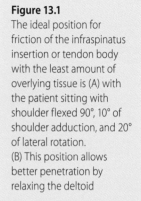

Figure 13.1
The ideal position for friction of the infraspinatus insertion or tendon body with the least amount of overlying tissue is (A) with the patient sitting with shoulder flexed 90°, 10° of shoulder adduction, and 20° of lateral rotation.
(B) This position allows better penetration by relaxing the deltoid

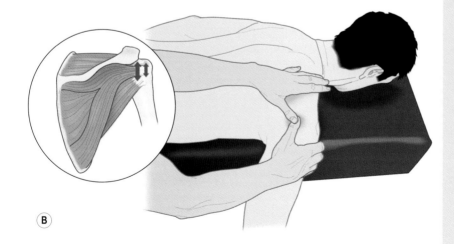

treatment of several sequences over several visits, if there are still functional tests that create pain at the CP, consider the PP.

A common knee injury is an acute sprain of the medial collateral ligament (MCL), which may end up as a chronic ache over the area. FM analysis would be beneficial regarding the coordination of the

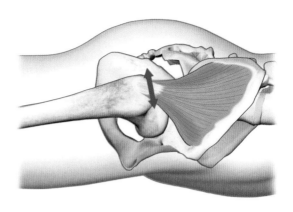

Figure 13.3
Gluteus medius at its insertion on the lateral surface of the greater trochanter. This is a treatment area for chronic trochanteric bursitis or tendinopathy

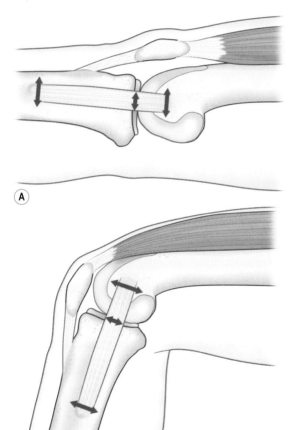

Figure 13.2
Medial collateral ligament. A sprain of this ligament should be frictioned at the most tender site during maximum allowable extension and flexion

lower extremity including the hip, pelvis, or foot, depending on the patient's history. But in an acute or especially chronic MCL sprain, treatment of the PP could prove to be essential for the complete manual treatment of the problem. Palpating for MCL involvement includes palpating and treating the most tender location found anywhere along this ligament (Figure 13.2). Other common (PP) areas of local pathology that respond to local friction can be a gluteus medius tendinosis or bursits (Figure 13.3), tested by the resisted lateral abduction of the gluteus medius. An acromioclavicular (A-C) joint is usually painful on passive shoulder abduction from 90° to 180° or horizontal shoulder adduction. Treatment would be localized over the A-C ligament (Figure 13.4). A common source of pain is over the supraspinatus insertion (Figure 13.5), tested specifically with patient's shoulder abducted to 90°, between the anterior and lateral plane with thumb up (Figure 13.6). All tendon insertions, myotendinous areas, and muscle bellies can be treated based on pathological reasons.

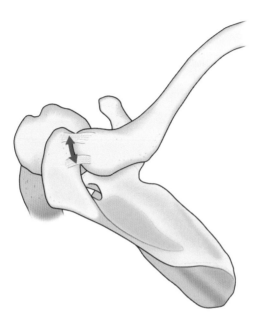

Figure 13.4
Acromioclavicular ligament (superior view). Friction should be applied with the forefinger along the joint line. The angle of the acromioclavicular joint can be variable

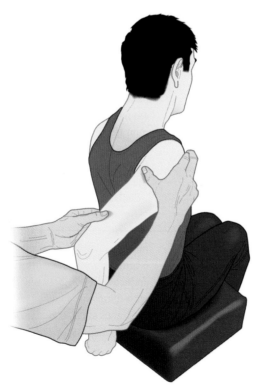

Figure 13.5
Supraspinatus. For maximum exposure of the supraspinatus insertion the patient's shoulder should be placed in maximal hyperextension, adduction, and medial rotation. Palpation should include anterior and anterior lateral area just below the humeral head including the greater tuberosity

Differentiating a pathological from a functional point: potential treatment modifications

Warren I. Hammer

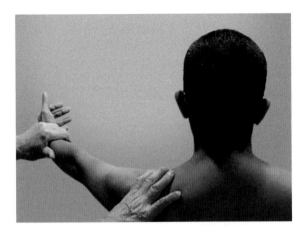

Figure 13.6
Testing the supraspinatus. Patient's shoulder abducted to 90°, between the anterior and lateral plane with thumb up

CASE REPORT

History

A 49-year-old executive who plays tennis twice a week complains of left shoulder pain for the past 2 months. He is right-handed. The patient states that his left shoulder aches almost constantly, especially with pain on abduction to 90°. He states that 5 years ago he was operated on his right shoulder for a full thickness tear of his supraspinatus. His right shoulder is 'painless.' He complains of intermittent cervical pain for 10 years. Absolutely no previous trauma or complaint of upper extremities, trunk or lower extremities. MRI revealed insertional tendinosis of left supraspinatus and arthritis of A-C joint.

Hypothesis

Evaluate cervical (CL), both shoulders (since left shoulder might be compensating for possible remaining post-surgical right shoulder fascial disruption), and scapular segment.

Table 13.1 Palpated points (PaVe)				
la-hu lt	me-hu lt	la-sc lt	me-sc lt	la-cl bi

Movement verification (MoVe)

In FM, from 1 to 3 asterisks are used to indicate pain, limited range of movement (ROM), or weakness. Results of MoVe: pain on left resisted abduction in the scapular plane (see Figure 13.6) (***), and pain with resisted left humeral abduction at 120° (frontal plane) testing (**). A painful arc was present on active and/or passive left shoulder abduction in all planes between 80° and 120° (**). A painful arc is active or passive arm elevation in either the sagittal, coronal or scapular planes. There is no pain from 60° to 80°, pain to about 120° and then no pain. This test represents pinching of structures in the subacromial space. Passive shoulder abduction from 90° to 180° (A-C joint was painful (**). Limited right lateral bending of cervical (CL) spine. Right shoulder, free painless ROM and normal with resisted and passive testing.

Palpation verification (PaVe)

On the left, densified and painful functional points (CCs) were found, as detailed in Table 13.1.

Pathological (PP): supraspinatus capsular insertion and A-C ligament (see Figure 13.4).

Treatment

On the first visit, only functional points listed in Table 13.1 were treated with FM. The supraspinatus test improved from (***) to (+). Resisted humeral abduction at 120° improved from (**) to (+), the painful arc improved from (**) to (+). A–C abduction test remained the same (**). Note: in FM, plus signs are used to indicate improvement.

2nd visit

One week later, some of the FM frontal plane points were re-treated, including la-di on the left and bilateral cervical FM points. All tests reached a (+++) except for the supraspinatus (+) and A–C ligament (**) tests. A–C ligament

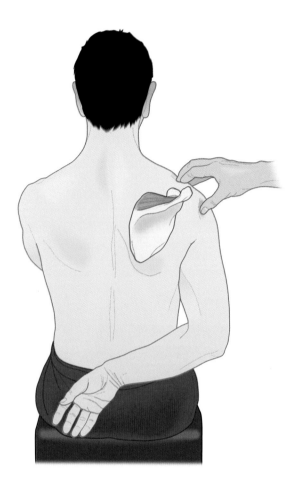

Figure 13.7
Treatment area of supraspinatus. Superior view of the supraspinatus insertion area located inferior to the anterior acromion, just proximal to the greater tuberosity

continued to be painful on palpation. Only pathological points A–C ligament (Figure 13.4) and supraspinatus tendon insertion (Figure 13.7) were treated for the 3rd and 4th visit. The patient was discharged after the 4th visit (+++).

Conclusion

It is hypothesized, based on other manual medicine methods over the years, that the site of tissue pathology may require treatment. The inclusion of the treatment of pathological points may enhance results obtained by using FM.

Hypothesis II

The retro-medio diagonal (that runs from the sacrum to the cervical region) represents both a functional and pathological pathway that should be assessed and probably treated for back pain even though it may not have been identified as a primary altered structure during FM assessment.

Hypothesis II infers that with spinal pain, a pathological area may exist, namely the multifidi muscles beneath the retro-medio (re-me) diagonal. Evidence exists that this muscle is directly associated with most back pain and should never be ignored during an FM evaluation for spinal pain. It is hypothesized that since the re-me diagonal covers the multifidi sequence, a change is required in the FM assessment protocol regarding this line. No matter which of the myofascial units, including diagonals and spirals, might appear primary in back pain, the re-me diagonal should be evaluated and treated.

Anatomically, the multifidus is made up of superficial and deep fibers. The superficial fibers have up to five fascicles that arise from the spinous processes and lamina of each lumbar vertebra and descend in a caudolateral direction to the transverse processes of three or more segments below (Macintosh et al. 1986). In the lumbar area, the superficial fascicles attach to the ilia and sacrum. The deep fibers attach from the inferior border of a lamina and insert into a mammillary process and facet joint capsule. There are no rotatores muscles in the lumbar or cervical area making the multifidi fibers the deepest in both areas. The superficial fibers are more distant from the center of rotation of the lumbar spine and have a moment arm for lumbar extension and control of lumbar lordosis while the deep fibers are near the center of lumbar rotation and are working throughout spinal ranges of motion (Moseley et al. 2002). The superficial multifidi contribute to the control of spine orientation. The deep fibers are thought to be active in all directions to modulate spinal compression for control of intervertebral shear and rotation forces. The deep fibers stabilize the vertebral joints at each level and control intersegmental motion. They provide stiffness and stability making each vertebra work more effectively and reduce the degeneration of the joint structures caused by friction from normal physical activity (Moseley et al. 2002) (Figure 13.8).

From an FM point of view

- Based on the action of the multifidi, bilateral backward extension, unilateral side-bending to the ipsilateral side and rotation to the contralateral side, treatment of this myofascial diagonal can relieve any of these motions. According to L. Stecco and A. Stecco (2017), 'unsynchronized activity of any paravertebral muscle can cause friction or conflict between vertebral joint facets because these muscles all contain fibers that act on the three spatial planes: if fibers on both sides of the vertebral column

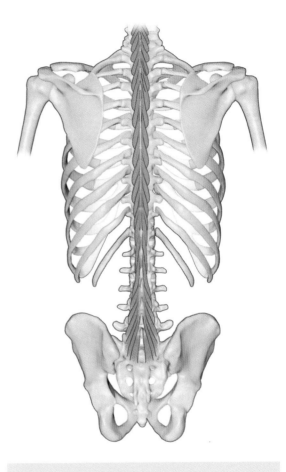

Figure 13.8
Illustration of multifidi

are activated, then they are extensors; if fibers on only one side are activated, then they are lateral flexors and if the oblique fibers are activated they are external rotators. Each group of fibers is connected with different portions of the fascia. Densification of one of these areas within the lumbar fascia causes incoordination between the muscle fibers resulting in joint conflict.'

- The cervical multifidi have muscle spindles, which are found predominantly as single units concentrated closely to the vertebral lamina (Boyd-Clark et al. 2002).

- Only the multifidi muscle bellies and interspinales have their own clearly defined fascial compartments while the rest of the erector spinae muscles are fused together (Stecco C. 2015).

- Reduced proprioception is reported in patients with low back pain as compared to control groups (Danneels et al. 2002).

- Given that in the neutral position, the head is maintained in slight flexion, the organization of spindles in the multifidus may be important for resisting gravitational forces that would otherwise encourage multifidus lengthening (Danneels et al. 2002).

- Chronic low back pain displayed significantly decreased multifidus muscle activity as compared to healthy subjects during coordination exercises, indicating that over the long term, back pain patients have a reduced ability to voluntarily recruit the multifidi muscles in order to maintain a neutral spine position (Danneels et al. 2002).

From a pathological (PP) point of view

- Trunk muscles have a limited ability compared to the deep multifidi that control intervertebral shear and tension by creating intervertebral compression. This ability to take pressure off the vertebral discs allows our body weight to be better distributed along the spine. EMG activity of all trunk muscles begins before the onset of upper or lower limb movement (Moseley et al. 2002).

- Multifidus degeneration, including reduced volume, increased fatty infiltration, and bilateral muscle asymmetry, has an association with degenerative lumbar spinal stenosis (Hodges et al. 2015).

- Multifidus muscle changes after back injury are characterized by structural remodeling of muscle, adipose, and connective tissue (Hodges et al. 2015).

- A study aimed at examining the association of low back pain (LBP) with muscle stiffness by using ultrasonic shear wave elastography and muscle mass of the lumbar back muscle, and spinal alignment in young and middle-aged medical workers found that LBP was associated with muscle stiffness of the lumbar multifidi muscles (Masaki et al. 2017).

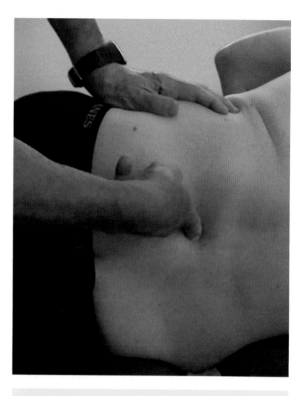

Figure 13.9
Palpation of the retro-medial line with the patient in a side/oblique position

- Preoperative MRI of the lumbar multifidi muscles that shows cross-sectional area atrophy can reliably be used to predict poorer postoperative outcomes following lumbar spinal decompression surgery (Zotti et al. 2017).

Discussion for hypothesis II

Palpation of re-me is usually performed on a prone patient, but in the lumbar area could also be treated with the patient in a side/oblique position (Figure 13.9).

Palpation usually reveals a nodular-like painful sensation especially since the deep fibers insert into a mammillary process and facet joint capsule. The pathological element compared to the functional element would indicate that a painful area is as important as a densification. Palpation of softness or depression may indicate a multifidus

Differentiating a pathological from a functional point: potential treatment modifications

Warren I. Hammer

deficit requiring multifidi exercises. In the lower lumbar area, it is necessary to palpate deeper due to the presence of deep adipose tissue. Most localized chronic spinal pain areas, for example in the thoracics, even though there is no history of cervical or lumbar involvement, require evaluation and treatment of proximal and distal spinal re-me locations. A frequent complaint is localized pain at the treatment site, for example at a particular re-me-lu, thoracic, or cervical area. Since these areas are regarded as both pathological (PP) and functional (FM) points, any of the painful re-me points may be involved. Some points may require over 5–10 minutes of treatment. It appears that in this myofascial diagonal, releasing a proximal point does not necessarily free up a distal point and vice versa.

Kader et al. (2000) found a correlation between atrophied lumbar multifidi and leg pain. However, the relationships between muscle atrophy and radiculopathy symptoms, nerve root compression, herniated nucleus pulposus and a number of degenerated discs were statistically not significant. They state that this may explain referred leg pain in the absence of other MRI abnormalities.

Conclusion

The special function and pathology of the multifidi muscles and their relation to back pain place the re-me myofascial diagonal in a different category than other myofascial diagonals or sequences. Regardless of the primacy of other sequences, for local and radiating spinal pain, re-me should always be considered.

References

Abate M, Silbernagel KG, Siljeholm C, Di Iorio A, De Amicis D, Salini V, Werner S and Paganelli R (2009) Pathogenesis of tendinopathies: Inflammation or degeneration? Arthritis Research and Therapy 11 (3) 235.

Boyd-Clark LC, Briggs CA and Galea MP (2002) Muscle spindle distribution, morphology, and density in longus colli and multifidus muscles of the cervical spine. Spine 27 (7) 694–701.

Danneels LA, Coorevits PL, Cools AM, Vanderstraeten GG, Cambier DC, Witvrouw EE and De CH (2002) Differences in electromyographic activity in the multifidus muscle and the iliocostalis lumborum between healthy subjects and patients with sub-acute and chronic low back pain. European Spine Journal 11 (1) 13–19.

Fede C, Albertin G, Petrelli L, Sfriso MM, Biz C, De Caro R and Stecco C (2016) Expression of the endocannabinoid receptors in human fascial tissue. European Journal of Histochemistry 60 (2) 2643.

Hammer WI (1991) Functional soft tissue examination and treatment by manual methods. Gaithersburg, MD: Aspen Publishers.

Hodges PW, James G, Blomster L, Hall L, Schmid A, Shu C, Little C and Melrose J (2015) Multifidus muscle changes after back injury are characterized by structural remodeling of muscle, adipose and connective tissue, but not muscle atrophy: Molecular and morphological evidence. Spine 40 (14) 1057–71.

Kader DF, Wardlaw D and Smith FW (2000) Correlation between the MRI changes in the lumbar multifidus muscles and leg pain. Clinical Radiology 55 (2) 145–9.

Loghmani MT and Warden SJ (2009) Instrument-assisted cross fiber massage accelerates knee ligament healing. Journal of Orthopaedic and Sports Physical Therapy 37 (7) 506–14.

Lundon K (2007) The effect of mechanical load on soft connective tissues, in WI Hammer (ed) Functional soft-tissue examination and treatment by manual methods, 3rd edn. Sudbury, MA: Jones and Bartlett, pp 33–161.

Macintosh JE, Valencia F, Bogduk N and Munro RR (1986) The morphology of the human lumbar multifidus. Clinical Biomechanics (Bristol, Avon) 1 (4) 196–204.

Masaki M, Aoyama T, Murakami T, Yanase K, Ji X, Tateuchi H and Ichihashi N (2017) Association of low back pain with muscle stiffness and muscle mass of the lumbar back muscles, and sagittal spinal alignment in young and middle-aged medical workers. Clinical Biomechanics (Bristol, Avon) 49 128–33.

Moseley GL, Hodges PW and Gandevia SC (2002) Deep and superficial fibers of the lumbar multifidus muscle are differentially active during voluntary arm movement. Spine 27 (2) E29–E36.

Ombregt L, Bisschop P and Veer HJ (2003) A system of orthopedic medicine, 2nd edn. Philadelphia: Churchill Livingstone.

Pavan PG, Stecco A, Stern R and Stecco C (2014) Painful connections: Densification versus fibrosis of fascia. Current Pain and Headache Reports 18 (8) 441.

Stecco C (2015) Functional atlas of the human fascial system. Edinburgh: Churchill Livingstone, Elsevier.

Stecco L and Stecco A (2016) Fascial manipulation for internal dysfunctions: Practical part. Padua: Piccin.

Stecco L and Stecco A (2017) Fascial manipulation for musculoskeletal pain: Theoretical part, 2nd edn. Padua: Piccin.

Zotti MGT, Boas FV, Clifton T, Picche M, Yoon WW and Freeman BJC (2017) Does pre-operative magnetic resonance imaging of the lumbar multifidus muscle predict clinical outcomes following spinal decompression for symptomatic spinal stenosis? European Spine Journal 26 (10) 2589–97.

Postural changes after three treatments in patients with chronic cervical pain

Lorenzo Copetti, Italy

14

EDITOR'S COMMENT

Rather than a single case report, this chapter presents a randomized clinical pilot study concerning the application of Fascial Manipulation®–Stecco® (FM) method in patients with measurable postural alterations due to chronic neck pain (CNP). In particular, the author, who has more than 20 years of experience with this method, has used computerized dynamic platform posturography to measure postural changes before and after three treatments in 12 women with CNP, with a follow-up at 3 months. This study discusses how this manual method, which aims at restoring normal fascial tension throughout the body, may improve peripheral proprioceptive input, enhancing postural stability and control over time. According to each patient's history and concomitant symptoms, treatments involved both the Fascial Manipulation for Internal Dysfunctions (FMID) approach and the musculoskeletal approach. While individual points treated in each treatment are not reported here due to the number of patients involved, this chapter is an example of how the impact of FM on specific parameters can be examined in detail.

Author's background

Since graduating as a physiotherapist (Udine, Italy) in 1981, I have always worked in private practice with a predominately musculoskeletal caseload that has more recently also included internal dysfunctions. Over the years, the methods I have studied and applied include Bricot's posturology, Cyriax's deep transverse massage, osteopathic techniques, Global Postural Re-education by Souchard and Visceral Manipulation by Barral. Between 1992 and 2016 I taught a manual therapy course at what was initially a regional school for physiotherapists, and subsequently became part of the physiotherapy degree course at the University of Udine, Italy.

Experience with Fascial Manipulation®– Stecco® method

I first started studying Fascial Manipulation®–Stecco® method (FM) in 1997, at one of the first courses that Luigi Stecco taught in Italy, because I was looking for more lasting results as compared to the techniques I already used. At that stage, 16 years into my career, I had noticed that while I was able to run a successful practice and certainly help a large number of patients to have some relief, I saw some people who returned over and over again, either with the same symptoms or different symptoms, but always apparently related to the presenting problem.

In the beginning, it was not easy to assimilate the new concepts proposed by Luigi Stecco. My previous work focalized treatment more or less locally with respect to symptoms, and it was difficult to accept that the origin of a problem could arise from another part of the body, often at a significant distance from the symptom. I had already developed some understanding of distantly related areas by incorporating a deep massage according to Shizuto Masunaga (Masunaga & Ohashi 1977), a Japanese psychologist and shiatsu master who introduced a new interpretation of classical meridians, into my own personal combination of techniques. However, at most I was treating the antagonist muscle to resolve a problem in the agonist muscle.

Over time I realized that Luigi's proposals, which were being continuously improved, represented the answers I was looking for, offering lasting results for the myofascial-skeletal system as a whole. Although FM initially seems rather simple – a series of fascial points to work on in a pattern – the need to interpret each individual patient and understand their unique patterns of compensations makes it more difficult than it first seems. Nevertheless, my increasing capacity to apply Luigi's proposals, together

CHAPTER 14

with his almost monthly updates and the scientific evidence that started to sustain the basic principles of the method itself, all contributed to achieving better and lasting results. Even though I have been a certified teacher of FM since 1998 I still continue to study the myofascial system every day.

In the first 3 or 4 years of practicing this method, my skepticism and curiosity led me to integrate these proposals with the other techniques I was more familiar with. In particular, I used postural analysis based on Posturology by Bricot (1999) and forms of osteopathic analysis to evaluate patients before and after FM treatments, and I often added high velocity manipulations to complete the work started with FM. However, as I became more competent in identifying correlated densifications within fascial structures, the less I needed to apply other techniques to complete the treatment.

While I presently recognize that FM may not always be the only approach required to resolve the problems that every patient presents, it is certainly a mainstay in my clinical reasoning and I constantly use the FM evaluation as part of my initial screening process. My experience has shown that balancing the fascial system and rendering it efficient is a necessary baseline for other approaches, such as proprioceptive re-education, muscle reinforcement and motor pattern retraining or even pain management, all of which may be necessary to different degrees according to the patient's individual situation.

CASE REPORT

Postural changes after three treatments of Fascial Manipulation®–Stecco® method in 10 patients with chronic cervical pain

Introduction

The capacity for human beings to maintain postural balance has been a topic that has fascinated me ever since I first started to study physiotherapy. I have to thank one of my teachers, Professor Francesco Mariotto, for this passion. His curiosity towards all aspects concerning maintenance of posture and how rehabilitation could improve postural control, particularly in subjects with scoliosis, have been an inspiration. When I started studying posture in the 1970s, it seemed certain that the central nervous system (CNS), together with the cerebellum and the reticular formation of the brainstem, was entirely responsible for postural control.

Nevertheless, information was emerging that peripheral structures, such as receptors within the muscles and tendons, could also have an important role in postural balance control. Needless to say, at that time no mention was ever made of fascia, fascial tissues or even connective tissues as having a potential role in postural balance feedback mechanisms.

My part-time university teaching position also involved collaborating with students in the final year of their physiotherapy degree course, mentoring them and supervising their degree theses. Over the years I have supervised theses dealing with FM treatments for carpal tunnel syndrome (2000), painful shoulder in hemiplegic adults (2004), fibromyalgia (2013), and overactive bladder dysfunction (2013), as well as several theses about changes that can be measured after FM treatment using instruments such as surface electromyography, an isokinetic device, ultrasonography and elastography (2007; 2009; 2015).

Given my passion for postural balance and control, when a student proposed a study for his physiotherapy degree thesis concerning the possible effects of FM on postural balance in subjects with chronic neck pain (CNP), I accepted with enthusiasm. In particular, the study involved the evaluation of post-treatment changes in the upright posture utilizing computerized dynamic platform posturography, which allowed for an accurate recording of even small variations in postural balance.

Already in the late 1990s, Gagey and Weber (1997) and Bricot (1999) had demonstrated that the maintenance of the upright position involves continuous oscillations on the frontal and sagittal planes. Gagey and Weber

Postural changes after three treatments in patients with chronic cervical pain

Lorenzo Copetti

maintained, however, that because the amplitude of these oscillations is not sufficient to stimulate the cerebellum or the vestibular apparatus, there has to be another mechanism that is involved in the registration and correction of postural balance. More recent studies of the innervation of the fascia (Stecco C. et al. 2007; Tesarz et al. 2011), together with a greater understanding of the complexity of the fascial system architecture itself (Stecco C. 2015), suggest that deep muscular fascia could have proprioceptive properties, which may represent the mechanism that Gagey hypothesized. In effect, the fasciae link proprioceptive elements such as the deep neck muscles, which are rich in proprioceptors and muscle spindles, to the eyes and the labyrinths, permitting accurate processing of sensory information in order to regulate head position and balance. Grgić (2006) suggests that mechanoreceptors within cervical intervertebral joints, deep cervical fasciae, ligaments, and muscle spindles located in the deep, short muscles of cervical spine form a so-called cervical proprioceptive system (CPS). Yet other authors (Yahia et al. 2009) link impaired cervical proprioception and neck movement limitations in CNP to the extensive anatomical connections between neck proprioceptive input and vestibular input. Furthermore, patients with CNP have a significant increase in the thickness of their cervical fascia as compared to a control group without chronic pain (Stecco A. et al. 2014a). In particular, thickness of the loose connective tissue layers is greater than the fibrous sublayers and this could correlate to a perception of stiffness coupled with an altered dynamic response of the mechanoreceptors embedded within the fascia, causing pain and alteration in proprioception.

Traditionally, the acquisition of any given 'static' posture is determined by a voluntary act that is initiated in the CNS. To bring about movement, the CNS impulse tensions the muscle spindles via the gamma fibers, which, in turn, activate the extrafusal fibers by means of the alpha motoneuron. Once the desired posture or position has been obtained, it is maintained via the contraction of muscles in response to any minimal loss of balance or equilibrium. These muscles are activated via the spinal circuit in response to minute stretches of the muscle spindles.

L. Stecco (2004) underlines the fact that muscle spindles are inserted within the perimysium of the fascia and, therefore, the fascia has to be functionally and structurally integral in order to allow muscle spindles to fire in an optimal manner. Furthermore, he suggests that the tone of the muscle fibers that insert directly onto fascia (approximately 35–40% of muscle fibers in each muscle) contributes to maintaining a receptive network that is sensitive to even minute variations in length. According to A. Stecco et al. (2014b), any alteration within muscular fascia could potentially interfere with muscle spindle functioning, generating an altered response of the CNS with regards to posture maintenance. The consequent alteration in the posture itself, however, would be perceived as being 'normal', leading to an imbalance in muscular activity, that, over time, could produce a variety of symptoms.

Different authors report changes in muscle recruitment postural sway and postural instability in patients with neck pain due to whiplash (Ruhe et al. 2011; Juul-Kristensen et al. 2013) indicating the presence of disturbed sensory feedback patterns in people with whiplash associated disorders. Interestingly, a systematic review by Silva and Cruz (2013) suggests that both patients with idiopathic neck pain and those with whiplash-associated disorders have poorer balance than healthy controls.

Hypothesis

It was hypothesized that applications of FM, a manual therapy aimed at restoring fascial equilibrium, in patients with chronic neck pain and whiplash-associated disorders could affect postural control in these subjects. Due to the extended period of time that fascial alterations may have been present, also possibly in segments other than the neck region, it was predicted that postural changes would not necessarily be evident immediately after treatment but would require a period of time for eventual proprioceptive changes to be integrated into movement control. Through restoring tensional balance within the fascial system, predicted pain reduction and subsequent increased range of movement would have contributed further to improving postural control.

CHAPTER 14

Methodology

Eighteen female subjects with a history of chronic cervical pain lasting more than 3 months, including sequels from whiplash-associated disorders, were recruited from a waiting list for physiotherapy care at the department of rehabilitative medicine at the Gervasutta Hospital, Udine, Italy, and randomized into a study group (A) with 12 participants (39.75 years; DS 8.2) and a control group (B) with 6 participants (32.5 years; DS 4.23).

Inclusion criteria:

- age between 18 and 50 years
- evident limitation in range of movement of the cervical segment
- at least 3 months of cervical pain, including whiplash associated disorders.

Exclusion criteria:

- undergoing other physical therapy or pharmacological treatments that could potentially influence the results of the FM treatment
- concomitant pathologies, e.g., neurological, rheumatological disorders
- previous cervical vertebra fracture
- marked cervical arthroses with osteophytes.

Group A received three weekly sessions of FM over a total period of 21 days. Each subject in group A was evaluated prior to and after every treatment session and at 3 months after they had concluded their treatments (T7) (Table 14.1). Group B received no treatment and this group was re-evaluated 3 months (T7) after the initial evaluation (T1).

Evaluations

On entry (T1) all patients were evaluated for:

1. pain measured on a visual analog scale (VAS)
2. range of active neck movements (ROM) utilizing the Bioval system (produced by RM Ingénierie). The Bioval consists of software and a series of inertial wireless sensors within one or more motionpods that are attached to the body in order to measure kinematic movements of the body segments in the three planes of space without limiting freedom of movement. The sensors within each motionpod transmit data at the rate of 30 measurements per second to a computer where they are then translated onto a cartesian system of reference. Six active movements of the neck segment, including flexion, extension, lateral flexion to the left and right, and rotation to the left and right, were evaluated in all patients by the Bioval sensors that were attached to frontal region, the spinous process of the fifth thoracic vertebra and on the lateral side of the face, just in front of the ear. For these movements, subjects were all in the seated position,

Table 14.1 Summary of treatment program for group A

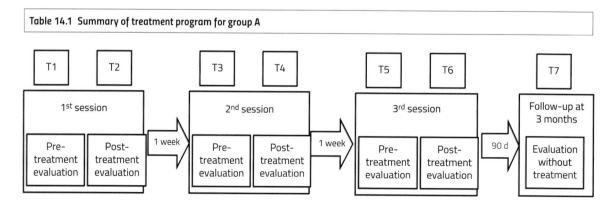

with back support, knees and hips flexed to 90°, feet resting on the floor, and hands resting on their thighs

3. postural sway in the upright position. This was measured by computerized dynamic platform posturography (CDPP). The apparatus used was a Pedoscan (Diers Medical systems, Inc) (Figure 14.1, Table 14.2), which captures and displays the pressure distribution on the human foot when the person is standing. High-frequency measurements (300 Hz) allow for rapid movements of the body's center of gravity and load changes to be recorded. The total excursion of the center of pressure (COP) along the sagittal and frontal axes was measured. The COP is the resultant of the trajectory of the center of mass and the amount of torque applied at the support surface to control body-mass acceleration. In other words, the COP is the center of the distribution of the total force applied to the supporting surface. The apparatus measures (in centimeters) the distance that the COP varies during the maintenance of posture over the time of the measurement (30 seconds) – fewer centimeters indicates more stability. This CDPP apparatus was connected to a computer via a USB cable and the DICAM version 2.1.0 program was used for data analysis.

Markings (Figures 14.2, 14.3) were applied to the platform in order to maintain uniformity in positioning throughout evaluation. Subjects were all barefoot and they were asked to maintain the standing position for 30 seconds with their eyes open.

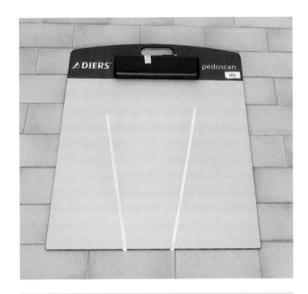

Figure 14.1
Computerized dynamic platform posturography: Pedoscan (Diers®)

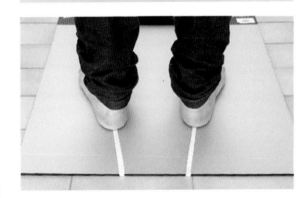

Figure 14.2
Positioning of the feet over markings, posterior view

Table 14.2 Technical data sheet: Pedoscan (Diers®)	
Pedoscan (Diers®) technical data sheet	
Number of sensors	4096
Dimension of the sensory surface	480 mm × 320 mm
Dimension of an individual sensor	7 mm × 5 mm
Sensitivity	0.27 N/cm² – 127 N/cm²

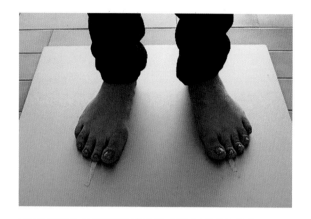

Figure 14.3
Positioning of the feet over markings, anterior view

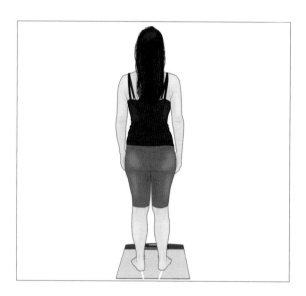

Figure 14.4
Full length view of the upright position on the platform

CDPP was performed before (T1, T3, T5) and after (T2, T4, T6) each treatment in group A, with a follow-up evaluation at 3 months (T7) after the conclusion of treatment. Group B was evaluated at T1 and T7. Patients (Figure 14.4) were blinded to the results of the data

throughout the CDPP evaluation procedures. All measurements were performed by G. Z.

FM treatments

The 12 patients in group A were all initially evaluated by L. C. according to the FM procedure, which includes an in-depth history taking with particular emphasis placed on previous traumas and/or any visceral dysfunctions. According to each person's history, additional segments, other than the neck segment, were selected for movement verification. Altered movements were noted for a post-treatment evaluation.

Comparative palpation verification of selected body segments was then performed in order to identify the altered fascial structure and FM treatments were performed on a weekly basis for 3 sessions.

Results

Group A

VAS: immediately after treatment (at T2/T4/T6): there was a mean reduction of 60.2% (2.1 points on the VAS scale).

Follow up at 3 months: there was a mean reduction of 52.1% (2.0 points on the VAS scale).

CDPP:

(Interpreting changes in center of pressure: a reduction in the total excursion of COP is indicative of an improvement (overall reduction in postural sway on sagittal and frontal planes) and an increase is considered to be indicative of a worsening of postural control.)

Immediately after treatment (mean of measurements at T2/T4/T6): 58.3% of evaluations presented a mean reduction in COP of 4.3% (9.6 cm) and 41.7% presented a mean increase in COP of 5.5% (11.2 cm), representing a mean decrease in COP of 0.2% (0.9 cm) between T2 and T6 (Figure 14.5).

Postural changes after three treatments in patients with chronic cervical pain

Lorenzo Copetti

Note: two subjects from group A received treatments between T6 and T7 that were not within this project and therefore they were excluded from the follow-up data. Follow-up at 3 months (T7): Mean reduction in COP of 11% (24.3 cm) for all subjects in group A. In particular, 80% (8/10) had a mean reduction of 14.7% (32.3 cm) and 20% (2/10) had mean increase in COP of 3.6% (7.6 cm) (Figure 14.6).

Active ROM: immediately after treatment (at T2/T4/T6) there was a mean increase in ROM of 8.7%.

Follow-up at 3 months: T1–7 there was a mean increase in active ROM of 23.7%.

Control group B

CDPP: between T1 and T7 there was a mean increase of 4.8% (9.5 cm) (Figure 14.7).

Active ROM: between T1 and T7 and mean increase in ROM of 3.2%.

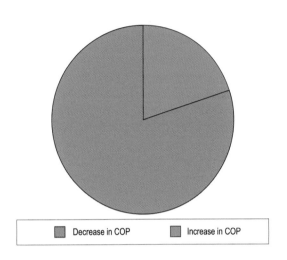

Decrease in COP   **Increase in COP**

Figure 14.6
Graph showing results of group A at T7 (3-month follow-up); 8/10 (80%) of patients in group A had a reduction in the center of pressure

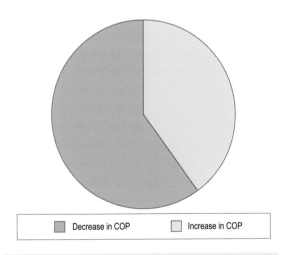

Decrease in COP   **Increase in COP**

Figure 14.5
Graph showing mean of center of pressure (COP) measurements at T2/T4/T6 (immediately after each treatment) in the study group A: 41.7% showed a mean increase in the COP and 58.3% had a mean reduction

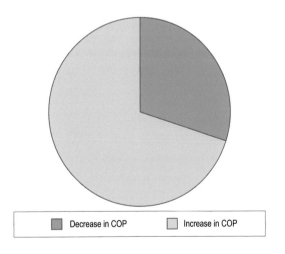

Decrease in COP   **Increase in COP**

Figure 14.7
Graph showing results of group B at T7 (3-month follow-up); 66.7% of patients in the control group B show an increase in the center of pressure (COP), compared to the 33.3% that show a reduction in the COP

Figure 14.8 is a graph that represents a comparison between the study group A and the control group B in terms of changes in the COP between T1 and T7.

Discussion

All subjects in this study were females. This was not an inclusion criterion but merely reflects the gender of patients who were seen at the department of rehabilitative medicine of the Gervasutta Hospital in the period of recruitment to this study; it nevertheless, gave homogeneity to the groups.

L. Stecco and C. Stecco (2009) emphasize the importance of analyzing previous fascial or tensional compensations as they could potentially influence the maintenance of posture. With regards to specifics of the FM evaluation, subjects presented various previous traumas that were not always comparable in terms of severity. The history of each individual patient was unique, as is commonly found in clinical practice. In some cases, the origin of the disturbance was related to previous whiplash associated disorders; in some it was apparently related to maladaptive work positions; in others there was an idiopathic onset. Nevertheless, the majority of cases had some history of previous trauma that was partially compensated.

During the FM assessment process, the choice of segments to examine with movement and palpation verification is always determined by the patient's individual history. Some subjects had concomitant internal disorders, such as painful menstrual cycles, gastritis, colitis, tachycardia, asthma, and panic attacks. In two cases, these symptoms were apparently isolated from the traumatic event, whereas in eight out of the 10 cases assessed at the 3-month follow-up, these symptoms had developed after the previous trauma, implicating a possible somato-visceral tensional compensation. In accordance with each patient's history and concomitant symptoms, treatment involved both the Fascial Manipulation for Internal Dysfunctions (FMID) approach and the musculoskeletal approach.

Prior to analyzing the results from the computerized dynamic platform posturography, the results concerning VAS measurements and neck movements in the study group A, will be considered in brief. A mean reduction in pain on the VAS scale immediately after each treatment (60%) was generally maintained at the 3-month follow-up (52%).

Initial small changes were seen in range of movement (ROM) after each treatment (8.7% overall) but this

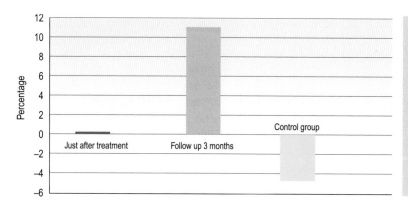

Figure 14.8
This diagram compares the changes in the center of pressure between T1 (at the beginning of treatment) and T7 (3-month follow-up) in the study group A (purple) and the control group B (yellow)

Lorenzo Copetti

improvement had increased at the 3-month follow-up (23.7%).

An immediate clinically significant reduction in pain could allow a more rapid return to normal movement, which then has long-term benefits in overall ROM. A somewhat similar outcome of statistically significant improvements in neck flexion ROM has been documented in another small clinical trial (Picelli et al. 2011) involving three applications of FM in subjects with whiplash-associated disorders. However, these results in ROM were measured at a 2-week follow-up and in our study an even greater improvement in ROM was seen after 3 months.

Interestingly, the results obtained from computerized dynamic platform posturography in the study group did not initially show clinically significant improvement; however, the long-term results at 3 months were definitely more positive. The immediate post-treatment variations were minimal and were possibly justifiable by the irritation of the fascia in the various segments that had been treated. This outcome had been predicted because if the muscular fibers and their relative fascia were in a disturbed state for an extended period of time then restoring correct functioning to the myofascial units would not have brought about an immediate recovery of the strength and the resistance of these structures. It was predictable that this recovery would have required a certain period of time for the integration of proprioceptive changes within a framework of reduced pain and it was hypothesized that improvement in proprioceptive input could have enhanced this recovery.

While two subjects in the control group (B) also had a reduction in the sway path of the COP at the 3-month follow-up (T7), it was significantly inferior to the changes that occurred in the study group (A). In effect at T7, the study group A had a mean reduction in COP of 11% (24.3 cm) while the control group had a general mean increase of 4.8% (9.5 cm).

Inaccurate or poorly integrated positional information from the vestibular system or neck proprioceptors could cause errors in CNS programming of head position. Furthermore, hypertonus of the neck muscles could increase mechanoreceptor activity resulting in confusion between impulses coming from the periphery, the vestibular system and other sensory systems involved in maintaining bodily balance. Consequently, inadequate vestibulospinal and vestibulo-ocular reactions and disturbances in reflex regulation of postural muscle tonus contribute to 'general instability.'

The improvement seen in group A could be explained by the restoration of correct gliding within the fascia that enhanced proprioceptive information and enabled correct functioning of muscular fibers during daily and sport activities.

Conclusion

Restoring correct fascial tension in subjects with CNP could permit better control of posture via improved interactions with the CNS. In subsequent studies it would be useful to add a functional scale, such as the short-form McGill Pain Questionnaire, in order to have a broader evaluation of pain, quality of pain, and functional improvements. Furthermore, given its role in postural control, modifications likely occurred also in the CNS, which suggests that further research could focus on dynamic magnetic resonance of the central areas involved in postural control in order to validate or confute this hypothesis.

Author's note

Many thanks to Gianluca Zannier, my former student and now physiotherapy colleague, who initiated this study.

CHAPTER 14

References

Bricot B (1999) La riprogrammazione posturale globale. Rome: Statipro – Marrapese.

Gagey PM and Weber B (1997) Posturologia: Regolazione e perturbazioni della stazione eretta. Rome: Marrapese.

Grgić V (2006) Cervicogenic proprioceptive vertigo: Etiopathogenesis, clinical manifestations, diagnosis and therapy with special emphasis on manual therapy. LijecVjesn 128 (9–10) 288–95.

Juul-Kristensen B, Clausen B, Ris I, Jensen RV, Steffensen RF, Chreiteh SS, Jørgensen MB and Søgaard K (2013) Increased neck muscle activity and impaired balance among females with whiplash-related chronic neck pain: A cross-sectional study. Journal of Rehabilitation Medicine 45 (4) 376–84.

Masunaga S and Ohashi W (1977) Zen Shiatsu: How to harmonize yin and yang for better health. Tokyo: Japan Pubns.

Picelli A, Ledro G, Turrina A, Stecco C, Santilli V and Smania N (2011) Effects of myofascial technique in patients with subacute whiplash associated disorders: A pilot study. European Journal of Physical and Rehabilitation Medicine 47 (4) 561–8.

Ruhe A, Fejer R and Walker B (2011) Altered postural sway in patients suffering from non-specific neck pain and whiplash associated disorder: A systematic review of the literature. Chiropractic and Manual Therapies 19 (1) 13.

Silva AG and Cruz AL (2013) Standing balance in patients with whiplash-associated neck pain and idiopathic neck pain when compared with asymptomatic participants: A systematic review. Physiotherapy Theory and Practice 29 (1) 1–18.

Stecco A, Meneghini A, Stern R, Stecco C and Imamura I (2014a) Ultrasonography in myofascial neck pain: Randomized clinical trial for diagnosis and follow up. Surgical and Radiologic Anatomy 36 (3) 243–53.

Stecco A, Stecco C and Raghavan P (2014b) Peripheral mechanisms contributing to spasticity and implications for treatment. Current Physical Medicine and Rehabilitation Reports 2 (2) 121–7. doi: 10.1007/s40141-014-0052-3.

Stecco C (2015) Functional atlas of the human fascial system. Edinburgh: Churchill Livingstone.

Stecco C, Gagey O, Belloni A, Pozzuoli A, Porzionato A, Macchi V, Aldegheri R, De Caro R and Delmas V (2007) Anatomy of the deep fascia of the upper limb. Second part: Study of innervation. Morphologie 91 (292) 38–43.

Stecco L (2004) Fascial manipulation for musculoskeletal pain. Padua: Piccin.

Stecco L and Stecco C (2009) Fascial manipulation: Practical part. Padua: Piccin.

Tesarz J, Hoheisel U, Wiedenhöfer B and Mense S (2011) Sensory innervation of the thoracolumbar fascia in rats and humans. Neuroscience 194 302–8.

Yahia A, Ghroubi S, Jribi S, Mâlla J, Baklouti S, Ghorbel A and Elleuch MH (2009). Chronic neck pain and vertigo: Is a true balance disorder present? Annals of Physical and Rehabilitation Medicine 52 (7–8) 556–67.

EDITOR'S COMMENT

Colleagues around the world often ask me if the Fascial Manipulation®–Stecco® (FM) method can be used with children and, in particular, neurological cases. The author of this chapter had extensive experience in neurological pediatric physiotherapy prior to studying this approach. Her attentive exploration of this method and its integration into her neurological pediatric work represent pioneering clinical observations that have contributed to the development of courses with a particular pediatric focus. In general, this chapter presents valuable insights for colleagues wanting to apply this method in this field. The author shares her observations regarding the effects of this method in terms of elasticity, agonist/antagonist coordination, proprioception and movement quality. She also discusses how FM can be used to treat pain and, at the same time, the strategies she has developed for applying a tendentially painful technique in these young patients. The case reported in this chapter addresses an example of a treatment of a 6-year-old girl with left-sided hemiplegia. The author stresses that FM is used in her practice principally as a means of preparing for active movement training.

Author's background

As a Neuro-Developmental Treatment (NDT/Bobath) physiotherapist with over 25 years' experience of working in neurological pediatric physiotherapy, I currently practice in a private, multidisciplinary center (Terapiakeskus Terapeija) that specializes in therapy for children and adults with special needs. My caseload ranges from newborns to adolescents, some of whom are severely disabled. I also work with locomotor disorders of different kinds in children, adults and young athletes. Having a wide interest in methods that focus on motor control and development in children, I have attended numerous courses in child neurology, as well as orthopedics, sports injuries and functional training for young athletes. Depending on the child and their family's needs, I integrate several different methods into my practice in order to promote optimal active function. In addition to the NDT/Bobath approach I have used Kinesio Taping®, functional training, vibration, mobilization and sensory preparation.

Experience with Fascial Manipulation®–Stecco® method

Having completed all three levels of Fascial Manipulation®–Stecco® method (FM) training, I find that this kind of approach does not contradict the methods I previously applied in any way. FM gives explanations to problems, such as stiffness that extends beyond muscular insertions, that my previous anatomical studies have not been able to explain. It also provides new, plausible explanations for the origin and distribution of pain. I have used FM with neurological pediatric patients since 2013, particularly as a way to prepare for movement, as well as to treat pain.

Initially, the hardest part of applying FM with these patients was the evaluation. Most of my patients, apart from some adolescents, cannot express their sensations and there is not necessarily any previous or concomitant pain. Nor can they perform the standardized FM movement tests, which require selective movements and control that these children either have not yet achieved or will never acquire. Therefore, to overcome this impasse, I have had to develop my own way to gather the necessary information. Given that I know most of my patients from the time they were newborn or toddlers, I base my anamnesis on my knowledge of the stress that their myofascial structures have been exposed to (e.g., overuse in incorrect movement patterns, disuse due to absence of active movements, operations, orthoses and aids, etc.). I use the part of movement or performance that requires improvement for my pre- and post-treatment movement test. My experience as an NDT/Bobath therapist also helps me in the analysis of incorrect movement patterns and their possible effect on fascia. Anamnesis and observation guides my selection of the segments to palpate. Taking into consideration the convergence of forces in certain areas of fascia, my practice suggests that several segments participating in the incorrect movement patterns should be examined. I take videos before and after treatment to evaluate outcomes.

The effects of FM treatment

The effects overlap one another but they can be summarized into the following four areas:

Elasticity

When first starting to use FM, the most immediate observable effect was the additional range of movement (ROM) obtained during preparation for active movements, such as hip and knee extension and supination. It also has a softening effect on scars. Normally hard to stretch areas, such as the palm, popliteal and calcaneal insertions, as well as some hypertonic muscles, respond quickly to FM. This method works especially well with adolescents, often causing less pain than stretching; however, it is also a good method for babies and toddlers. The youngest patient I have treated with FM was a 9-month-old girl who experienced pain when crawling; immediately after treatment, she was able to crawl without pain.

My observation, and also according to my patients and their parents, has been that the effect of FM lasts longer than stretching alone. I hypothesize that FM may make the difference by affecting the gliding between muscle/fascia interfaces and intrafascial layers, along myofascial sequences and in both directions on the treated plane and that, given the innervation present in these tissues, this improved gliding could also enhance proprioceptive feedback. Children affected by cerebral palsy usually lose flexibility as they are growing, however, neurological children who have repeatedly received FM treatments during growth seem to have less movement restrictions, suggesting that the inclusion of this method in their therapy could slow down loss of flexibility.

Agonist-antagonist coordination

FM also influences agonist-antagonist coordination, giving movements a better quality for a longer time. By applying FM in neurological children, it is possible to influence agonist-antagonist coordination in one segment and along extended parts of the myofascial sequence. Hypertonic muscles (and muscles active in incorrect movement patterns) are usually weak, as are their antagonists. Increased tone makes antagonist activity more difficult due to inhibition and resistance. This inappropriate activation of muscles reduces active voluntary movements and consequently, the strengthening of antagonists to hypertonic muscles is difficult and selective movements are difficult to achieve. The application of FM in the preparatory phase facilitates agonist and antagonist recruitment: the hypertonic muscle appears to glide more freely and antagonist activation is easier, decreasing the influence of hypertonia in controlled active movements.

Stecco (Stecco L. 2004; Stecco L. & Stecco A. 2017) proposes that due to the fascial attachments that exist between agonist and antagonist myofascial units, via intermuscular septa and muscle attachments to fascia, altering the tension of the deep fascia of the agonist myofascial unit can affect the tension of the antagonist myofascial unit. According to A. Stecco et al. (2014), muscle tone can be compromised by either reduced or increased activity of muscle spindles caused by reduced compliancy of connective tissue. Therefore, when treating hypertonic muscles, an inhibition of this overactive stretch induced stimulation could be occurring. Treating the antagonists to hypertonic muscles could potentially enable these muscles to contract more effectively.

Proprioception and quality of movement

FM appears to have short- and long-term effects on movement quality. The immediate observed effect is that it becomes easier for the child to learn new movements or to perform selective movements, such as selective ankle dorsiflexion or knee extension (in contrast to mass movements often seen in neurological patients). This can be achieved by using a combination of centers of coordination (CC) as well as centers of fusion (CF) in FM treatments.

Treatment of neurological pediatric patients

Nita Tolvanen

Positive effects on body control and better movement awareness throughout the whole body have also been observed; for example, when balancing on a moving surface. This is possibly due to enhanced stimulation of proprioceptors in correctly tensioned fascia (Stecco A. et al. 2011). When gliding of deep fascia is restored in CFs, which are mostly located around joints, proprioceptive information from mechanoreceptors that are embedded in this tissue could be facilitated (Stecco C. 2015), allowing the child to adapt and react more easily.

When used repeatedly, FM appears to influence proprioception even more widely. Over time, older children who have had numerous FM treatments, express their sensations regarding densification and pain more precisely. I hypothesize that, in the absence of disturbing densification in CCs, they experience the sensation of movement and postural control more easily. Furthermore, treatment of CFs presumably augments information received from joints (Stecco L. & Stecco A. 2017), reinforcing body awareness and allowing perception of smaller changes, enabling qualitatively better movements and enhancing weight bearing. This also influences the engram of movements.

Pain and FM

Children with cerebral palsy and other neurological disorders often experience various kinds of pain. Pain can be caused by:

- hypertonia (especially when it is asymmetrically distributed)
- surgery
- prolonged sitting and inability to change position as often as necessary.

In these cases, I have observed that children, and especially adolescents with cerebral palsy, have a good and rapid response to FM.

Interestingly, when working with this method in children with hypertonia I have observed that densification is often distributed more superficially. In such cases, I hypothesize that fascial tension is altered by the underlying hypertonic muscles via the numerous insertions of muscles onto fascia.

Rather than pain, these children often feel itching during treatment of densification. They also report pain closer to the CC than to the centers of perception (CP). Because of this apparently more superficial tension, I work lightly at the beginning of the manipulation (especially on CFs) and more deeply when the initial tension gives way. Children quickly learn that the pain/itching goes away in 1–2 minutes. They often play while I manipulate or we play guessing games to distract the child. This means that I often have to treat a child in sitting or standing, adapting my position to access the CC/CF more effectively.

Understanding the distribution of forces by myofascial connections helps to explain 'why' pain is felt in a certain area (e.g., why posterior knee pain can have its origin either further distally or proximally or on the antagonist sequence/diagonal) and where to treat. The question is always: Where is the disturbed gliding that impedes this anatomical structure?

To quote one adolescent patient: 'FM makes moving easier. There is less restriction in the tight (hypertonic) muscles and it is also easier to recruit the others (antagonists)' (hemiplegia, age 14, telling how ankle flexion feels).

Collaboration with team members

I cooperate with speech therapists in my multidisciplinary team. I have tried using FM to prepare for speech therapy, in particular, when dealing with eating difficulties. With these treatments, it is possible to reduce facial sensitivity, making opening and closing of the mouth and chewing easier, both when there is temporomandibular joint restriction due to structural anomalies and operations and when there is chronic non-use.

In summary, when applying FM in neurological children, practitioners should be aware that the anatomical location of a CC or a CF might shift a little, presumably because of anomalous movement patterns affecting the fascia from birth. Therapists might need to treat more points in several fascial structures than in cases of normal muscle tonus (e.g., several CFs around one segment and several segments participating in the incorrect pattern of movement). As incorrect movement patterns usually include components on all planes, I often use CFs and complement these points with CC points.

CASE REPORT

Improving agonist-antagonist coordination of dorsiflexion in a hemiplegic ankle

Introduction

A. is a 6-year-old girl who was born with left-sided hemiplegia. Muscle tonus is increased more in the lower left leg. The dominant movement pattern is flexion, adduction, internal rotation in the hip, flexion in the knee, and plantarflexion in the ankle, with the heel off the ground. The left leg is 1.5 centimeters shorter than the right, which affects the movement pattern as A. compensates for this difference. She currently has a 5 millimeter raise in her foot orthosis, with future plans to increase it as she grows. Previously, when the leg length difference was less, her movement patterns alternated between the above movement pattern and keeping her heel on the ground by adopting knee hyperextension while rotating her pelvis backwards. Muscle tonus in the trunk and upper limb is low. The upper limb has a general flexion movement pattern, with wrist pronation and flexion and muscle tonus increasing associatively from low to high.

The long-term aim of physiotherapy is to improve use of the left side, including weight bearing on both the left leg and arm. In particular, this means the ability to extend the knee and hip during stance phase while keeping the heel on the ground. The aim is also to obtain selective dorsiflexion in the ankle, initially in sitting and later in walking, which entails performing dorsiflexion with the knee almost straight.

Hypothesis

I know from previous treatments with this child that stretching alone can achieve full ROM in all segments. Prior to either stretching or FM, both hip and knee extension ROM is mildly decreased and ankle dorsiflexion with knee straight is quite limited. In this session, the first aim is to train for selective dorsiflexion in sitting. Once achieved, this transferable skill is to be applied to standing and walking, including weight bearing with the entire foot on the ground. As A. plays a lot on the floor and on the ground outside, the ability to squat with both heels on the ground is another aim. Selective dorsiflexion of the ankle, symmetrical squatting and good weight bearing requires elasticity of gastrocnemius, soleus, quadriceps, and hamstrings, which, to some extent, can be gained by stretching. It also requires good coordination between agonists and antagonists. I have tried to achieve this previously, using brief mechanical vibration on the dorsiflexors to stimulate function and sometimes lengthier vibration on ankle extensors to tire the hypertonic muscles, as well as brushing and Kinesio Taping® in different combinations. I have chosen to use FM in this session because I have observed that I can simultaneously influence and improve elasticity, agonist-antagonist coordination and quality of movement with this method.

Methodology

Following observation of incorrect movement patterns and consideration of the fascial structures affected by repetitive movements, palpation of CCs and CFs was carried out in the segments of genu (ge), talus (ta), and pes (pe) on the left.

Initial palpation verification highlighted definite densification in re-ge, re-la-ge 2, re-la-ta, re-la-pe, re-me-pe, an-ta, an-me-pe, an-pe and to a lesser degree in re-ta, an-ge, ir-ta and ir-pe.

Treatment of neurological pediatric patients

Nita Tolvanen

Treatment (Table 15.1)

Table 15.1					
Points treated	re-la-ta 1	re-la-ge 2	re-la-pe		an-me-pe 2,3
	an-la-pe 2, 3	re-me-pe1,2	re-ge	an-ta	an-pe

Results

Screenshots (Figures 15.1, 15.2, 15.3), taken from a video, illustrate the best dorsiflexion movement before and after the FM treatment. Post-treatment improvement in ROM and the selective movement quality can be noted, particularly in reduction of toe extensor overactivity, allowing for selective dorsiflexion effectuated by the ankle flexors, without compensation of toe extensors. Following treatment, squatting, standing and walking with the heel to the ground were all easier. Keeping the heel on the ground also permitted improvement in active hip and knee extension. Similar treatment in a different session have also produced comparable results (Figures 15.4, 15.5).

Discussion

The ability to perform a movement does not mean a child with neurological problems will use it. Therefore, it is essential to teach the child to use any new ability gained through FM treatment. In the case presented here, this method is used as a way to *prepare* for more active movements. Enhanced proprioceptive feedback is required to make feedforward and active movements easier. Something that translates to 'Hey, now I can do

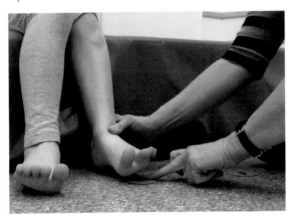

Figure 15.1
Best dorsiflexion before FM treatment. Frontal view. Not able to get ball of foot up with the heel on the ground. A lot of compensation with toe extensors in both feet

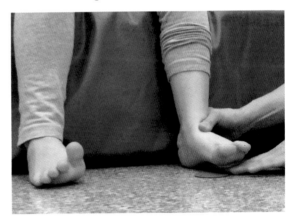

Figure 15.2
Best dorsiflexion after FM. Frontal view. Able to keep heel on ground and do a selective dorsiflexion without compensation of toe extensors

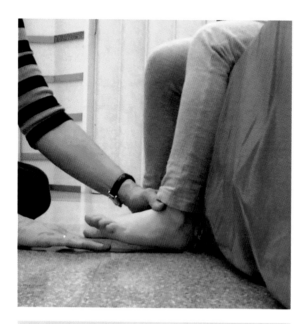

Figure 15.3
Best dorsiflexion after FM. Lateral view. Note the absence of compensation by toe flexors

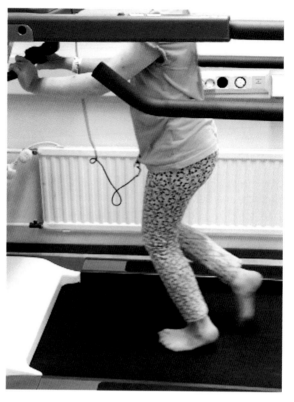

Figure 15.4
Screenshot from a video taken on another occasion after a long break from therapy; stance before FM

it and it feels like this.' Nevertheless, the integration of this new information into active movement does require extended, repetitive experience of that movement.

Evidence-based guidelines for clinical reasoning in such a specialized field as child neurology are limited. Clinical decisions have to rely on adult-based clinical research, as well as research regarding tissues and physiology. We need to consider that we work with children who are still developing and who have never learnt to move normally. Bar-On et al. (2015) underline that, in children who suffer from an early brain abnormality, spasticity is affected by the reorganization of supraspinal inputs and impaired motor maturation. This is very different to adults who have a developed locomotor system at the time of injury, such as a stroke. I think we also need to consider:

- the effects of the original damage in addition to other structural and functional problems

- individual factors, including motivation and understanding of the aims of therapy

- environmental factors, such as whether caretakers facilitate functional improvements, helping the child to use them.

Furthermore, hypertonus and spasticity are sometimes confused as being the same thing. In this chapter, the non-neural and neural factors in FM are discussed separately in reference to Bar-On et al.'s (2015) definition: hypertonus consists of neural (e.g., spasticity) and non-neural (e.g., soft tissue properties) factors affecting increased resistance to passive

Treatment of neurological pediatric patients
Nita Tolvanen

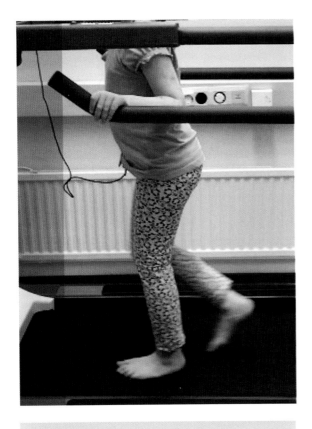

Figure 15.5
Screenshot from a video taken after FM treatment highlighting changes in stance on the left side

stretch in cerebral palsy. Bar-On et al. (2015) also underline that there is a difference between hypertonus in a resting muscle as compared to testing resistance to passive stretch (catch) and to hypertonia in active motion, which is difficult to evaluate. The word 'spasticity' is also used in the context of the above reference.

Clinical experiences of using FM in pediatric neurological physiotherapy as a way of preparing for active movement training are promising. Nevertheless, at present there is only one study (Raghavan et al. 2016) concerning the application of FM in neurological

patients (mostly adult stroke patients). In that study, hyaluronidase injections into CCs where used to treat spasticity in upper limbs. Hyaluronidase is an enzyme that hydrolyses hyaluronan (HA), a glycosaminoglycan that is abundant in deep muscular fascia and, when in a modified state, dramatically reduces the sliding movement of fascia (Cowman et al. 2015). The effects of hyaluronidase injections are similar to what is suggested happens during manual treatment of CCs and CFs, where friction induces a localized inflammatory process through an increase in tissue temperature. Raghavan et al.'s (2016) study demonstrated increased passive movements in all treated joints and increased active movements in most joints 2 weeks after the injection, with results being mostly maintained at a post-injection follow-up after 3 months. Also, muscle stiffness declined over time after the injection. Similar results were observed in the case study presented here: both passive and active movements were better and stiffness decreased. However, the manual effect lasts for a shorter time and the treatment has to be repeated.

Incorrect, repetitive and mostly invariable movement patterns affect extended fascial structures. When working with neurological patients, results are seldom achieved by treating only one segment. Raghavan et al. (2016) found that it was necessary to increase the number of muscles injected proximally and distally to the stiff muscle, along both the agonist and antagonist myofascial chains of the limbs. In my clinical experience, the need to treat along the affected myofascial sequence and on the antagonist sequence has been clear from the beginning, but the need to increase the number of muscles injected in Rhagavan's study somewhat confirms this clinical observation.

In the evaluation of A., palpation verification was performed in the left genu, talus, and pes segments. Coxa and pelvis segments were not palpated or treated since neither internal hip rotation nor pelvic tilting were currently problematic. The aim was to facilitate selective ankle dorsiflexion, an essentially sagittal plane movement but potentially affected by proprioceptive information also from CFs. Gastrocnemius was the most hypertonic muscle in the talus segment and treatment was applied both proximally (re-ge, re-la-ge) and distally (re-la-pe/re-me-pe) to this area, and also on the agonist myofascial chain (an-ta, an-pe, an-me-pe, an-la-pe). In particular, treatment of the very densified an-pe, located in the first metatarsal space, proved to be important in minimizing the compensation of poor dorsiflexion with extended toes.

Pavan et al. (2014) have shown that an interaction exists between hyaluronan (HA), lactic acid and alternations of pH in fascial tissue. The alteration of pH due to overuse, as occurs in spastic muscles, may also stimulate a reaction that increases HA viscosity, making muscles stiff (Stecco A. et al. 2013). Two very different studies (Stecco A. et al. 2014; Smith et al. 2011) have found that spasticity (hypertonus) affects the viscosity of extracellular matrix (ECM). Smith et al. (2011) focused on the increase in collagen fibers in the ECM and a lengthening of sarcomeres in spastic muscles, whereas A. Stecco et al. (2014) focused on the fact that the viscosity of ECM is due to an abnormal turnover of HA. Stecco (2014) suggests that high concentrations of HA cause alterations of connective tissue viscosity, affecting active muscle stiffness because of reduced gliding between layers of collagen fibers. Therefore, a manual technique, such as used in FM, that targets the ECM in densified muscular fascia merits further studies in neurological cases.

Bar-On et al. (2015) state that passive stiffness of the gastrocnemius-soleus and weakness of tibialis anterior are probably better predictors of limited dorsiflexion in terminal swing than spasticity. In the case study presented here, the aim was to increase elasticity in

gastrocnemius-soleus and to promote function of a weak tibialis anterior, compensated by overactive toe extensors. Selective dorsiflexion of the ankle emerged after FM® treatment but also better coordination in active movement when walking, squatting, and weight bearing dynamically on the left leg, with the heel on the ground during the stance phase of gait, and better extension of the knee.

These results could be explained by the possible effects of stiffer connective tissue on the neural components affected in spasticity. In the abovementioned article, Stecco et al. (2014) suggest that muscle spindles localized in perimysium have an important role in peripheral motor coordination and that increased stretch-induced stimulation of spindles in muscles with stiffer connective tissue could contribute to spasticity by reducing muscle spindle activation thresholds. Over-excitability of spindles can contribute to abnormal feedback and feed forward control of annulospiral endings (1ª afferents, sensory component), resulting in overactivation of alfa motor neurons that innervate the extrafusal muscle fibers (motor component). Furthermore, as antagonist muscle activity is inhibited by the stretch-reflex unit, any alteration in the regulation of agonist muscle tone can also affect antagonist activation.

Conclusion

Clinical experience of applying FM in pediatric neurological physiotherapy is proving to be promising. This approach is useful for preparing children for active movement training as it improves ROM and appears to balance agonist-antagonist activity, thereby enabling qualitatively better active movements and enhancing proprioceptive feedback.

Treatment of neurological pediatric patients
Nita Tolvanen

References

Bar-On L, Molenaers G, Aertbeliën E, Van Campenhout A, Feys H, Nuttin B and Desloovere K (2015) Spasticity and its contribution to hypertonia in cerebral palsy. BioMed Research International 2015: 317047. doi: 10.1155/2015/317047.

Cowman MK, Schmidt TA, Raghavan TA and Stecco A (2015) Viscoelastic properties of hyaluronan in physiological conditions. F1000Research 4: 622. doi: 10.12688/f1000research.6885.1.

Pavan PG, Stecco A, Stern R and Stecco C (2014) Painful connections: Densification versus fibrosis of fascia. Current Pain and Headache Reports 18 (8) 441. doi: 10.1007/s11916-014-0441-4.

Raghavan P, Ying L, Mircchandani K and Stecco A (2016) Human recombinant hyaluronidase injections for upper limb muscle stiffness in individuals with cerebral injury: A case series. EBioMedicine 9 306–13.

Smith L, Lee K, Ward S, Chambers H and Lieber R (2011) Hamstring contractures in children with spastic cerebral palsy result from a stiffer extracellular matrix and increased in vivo sarcomere length. Journal of Physiology 589 (P10) 2625–39. doi: 10.1113/jphysiol.2010.203364.

Stecco A, Stecco C, Macchi V, Porzionato A, Ferraro C, Masiero S and De Caro R (2011) RMI study and clinical correlations of ankle retinacula damage and outcomes of ankle sprain. Surgical and Radiologic Anatomy 33 (10) 881–90. doi:10.1007/s00276-011-0784-z.

Stecco A, Gesi M, Stecco C and Stern R (2013) Fascial components of myofascial pain syndrome. Current Pain and Headache Reports 17 352. doi: 10.1007/s11916-013-0352-9.

Stecco A, Stecco C, Raghavan P (2014) Peripheral mechanisms contributing to spasticity and implications for treatment. Current Physical Medicine and Rehabilitation Reports 2 2: 121–7. doi: 10.1007/s40141-014-0052-3.

Stecco C (2015) Functional atlas of the human fascial system. Edinburgh: Churchill Livingstone.

Stecco L (2004) Fascial manipulation for musculoskeletal pain. Padua: Piccin.

Stecco L and Stecco A (2017) Fascial manipulation for musculoskeletal pain: Theoretical part, 2nd edn. Padua: Piccin.

CONCLUSION

Once asked by a young colleague 'What is the most important ingredient for a practitioner of this method?', Luigi Stecco replied succinctly 'You need passion.' He then went on to explain how the passion for knowledge regarding the intricacies of fascial anatomy, including the musculoskeletal and visceral fascial systems, is necessarily the base ingredient for understanding and applying this approach.

The case reports in this book are just some examples of the wide-range of dysfunctions that can be treated using the Fascial Manipulation®–Stecco® (FM) method. Intended for practitioners who are commencing with this approach, as well as for other colleagues who are interested in knowing when this method can be applied, the actual treatment sections may be challenging for those who are unfamiliar with this method but they will hopefully stir curiosity.

Reading these case reports, one can find several emerging themes.

Firstly, the need to look beyond the presenting pain area to understand how dysfunction has installed itself in a patient. In particular, whenever a patient is complaining of pain without a clear cause, then the chronological order of past events, traumas, and surgery has to be considered carefully in order to understand how tensional compensations may have developed. Given that biarticular muscles and myofascial expansions connect the various body segments and insertional fasciae provide continuity between the musculoskeletal fasciae and the visceral fasciae, in accordance with presenting symptoms, the biomechanical models related to this method (see Introduction) can facilitate interpretation of any dysfunction within the fascial system.

Secondly, through the correct interpretation of these models, even chronic dysfunctions can often be resolved in a short number of sessions. Several contributors note that this clinical observation represented a turning point for them in terms of understanding the usefulness of this method.

Thirdly, the systematic analysis of each individual case can represent a challenge. The absence of protocols in this approach means that identifying key areas, the centers of coordination or fusion, can be a mentally demanding

process and the use of the method specific assessment chart is an essential element in this type of clinical reasoning. A completed assessment chart has not been presented with each case report for reasons of space; however, contributors consistently attest to its usefulness in their practice.

In effect, compilation of this assessment chart requires that the therapist engages the patient in an initial interview in order to collect details regarding the quality and characteristics of their presenting symptoms and the chronology of present and past events. This requires attentive listening skills and places the patient in the role of protagonist. The patient is normally informed of the therapist's hypothesis regarding their dysfunction prior to commencing an objective assessment, which consists of specific movement and palpation verifications. Interestingly, the entire procedure tends to enhance patient collaboration, allows the therapist to identify patient goals and any unhealthy belief systems, as well as creating an environment of trust where the patient perceives that their views are taken into consideration and that there is a logical treatment plan. These aspects permit the therapist to also consider social, emotional, cognitive, and psychological factors, which are all important issues, particularly when dealing with chronic pain patients.

Nevertheless, there is still a lot that has to be understood regarding the mechanisms by which working manually on soft tissue brings about changes in pain, postural alignment, muscle recruitment, and proprioceptive capacity. To date, the Stecco group has suggested that modifications of the extracellular matrix of fascial tissue, in particular, in the hyaluronan component within the loose connective tissue layers in key areas (centers of coordination and fusion) could be involved. Via traceable anatomical connections, these key areas appear to have specific tensional relationships as well as physiological relationships with muscle spindles, Golgi tendon organs, and the other innervation embedded within fasciae. It suggests that if the fascial tissue in these key areas is in an altered state, it can be modified by manual work, which raises the temperature of the tissue by means of friction and possibly sets off reactions either within the hyaluronan itself or by activating other receptors within the area, restoring the tissue to a physiological state. More recently, the Stecco group has also been investigating the role of endocannabinoid receptors in fascial tissue (Fede et al. 2016). McPartland (2008) first addressed this topic, suggesting that enhancement of endocannabinoid activity has extensive therapeutic potential for the treatment of somatic dysfunction, chronic pain, and neurodegenerative diseases, as well as inflammatory conditions, bowel dysfunctions, and psychological disorders. Fede et al. (2016) have demonstrated that the fibroblasts of the muscular fasciae express endocannabinoid receptors CB1 and CB2 and they suggest that the presence of these receptors could explain the role of fasciae as a pain generator and the efficacy of some fascial treatments by contributing to modulate fascial fibrosis and inflammation. In addition, with regards to internal dysfunctions, L. Stecco and C. Stecco (2013) present an interesting new hypothesis for the interaction between the internal and superficial fasciae and the autonomic system.

Could there be yet other mechanisms at play during treatment? Luigi Stecco emphasizes that the pressure used during comparative palpation should be such that it would not cause pain in normal tissue and that treatment pressure should be the minimum amount required to develop friction on the fascia (Stecco L. & Stecco A. 2017). Nonetheless, when friction is applied to altered soft tissue during treatment it can be painful for 2–3 minutes, and then the pain drops down dramatically (Borgini et al. 2010). Could 'pain inhibiting pain' mechanisms, within the broad category of heterotopic noxious conditioning stimulation (Sprenger et al. 2011), also be involved? Deep friction is generally applied to altered areas that are at a distance from reported painful

sites, indicating that there may also be a modulatory network, either within the spinal cord or directly via other central nervous structures, that relates the treatment sites with the reported painful sites.

Furthermore, prior to commencing treatment, patients are advised that these altered areas can be painful and they are instructed to report changes in pain levels as treatment proceeds. Patient expectancy regarding pain intensity and the efficacy of a painful technique as opposed to a non-painful technique could have an impact on treatment outcomes (Goffaux et al. 2007).

Stecco also emphasizes that selecting the correct pattern of altered centers of coordination and fusion is fundamental for effective treatment. While one pilot randomized clinical trial of sham treatments versus treatment according to FM guidelines in women with carpal tunnel syndrome (Pintucci et al. 2017) has indicated some positive short-term outcomes, the authors concluded that larger studies are warranted to distinguish the effects of the intervention from a placebo/analgesia effect.

In conclusion, if we can agree that clinical experience does have its own validity and importance within the evidence-based triad, then the popularity of FM among manual therapy practitioners in many different countries merits attention. The underlying mechanisms involved in its reported effectiveness are potentially manifold and offer multiple opportunities for further research.

References

Borgini E, Stecco A, Day JA and Stecco C (2010) How much time is required to modify a fascial fibrosis? Journal of Bodywork and Movement Therapies 14 (4) 318–25. doi: 10.1016/j.jbmt.2010.04.006.

Fede C, Albertin G, Petrelli L, Sfriso MM, Biz C, De Caro R and Stecco C (2016) Expression of the endocannabinoid receptors in human fascial tissue. European Journal of Histochemistry 60 (2) 2643. doi: 10.4081/ejh.2016.2643.

Goffaux P, Redmond WJ, Rainville P and Marchand S (2007) Descending analgesia—when the spine echoes what the brain

expects. Pain 130 (1–2) 137–43. doi:10.1016/j.pain.2006.11.011.

McPartland JM (2008) The endocannabinoid system: An osteopathic perspective. Journal of the American Osteopathic Association 108 586–600.

Pintucci M, Imamura M, Thibaut A, de Exel Nunes LM, Mayumi Nagato M, Kaziyama HH, Tomikawa Imamura S, Stecco A, Fregni F and Rizzo Battistella L (2017) Evaluation of fascial manipulation in carpal tunnel syndrome: A pilot randomized clinical trial. European Journal of Physical and Rehabilitation Medicine 53 (4) 630–1. doi: 10.23736/S1973-9087.17.04732-3.

Sprenger C, Bingel U and Büchel C (2011) Treating pain with pain: Supraspinal mechanisms of endogenous analgesia elicited by heterotopic noxious conditioning stimulation. Pain 152 (2) 428–39. doi:10.1016/j.pain.2010.11.018.

Stecco L and Stecco C (2013) Fascial manipulation for internal dysfunctions. Padua: Piccin.

Stecco L and Stecco A (2017) Fascial Manipulation® for musculoskeletal pain: Theoretical part, 2nd edn. Padua: Piccin.

INDEX

Note: Page number followed by f and t indicates figure and table respectively.

INDEX

INDEX

INDEX